Workbook of Diagnostics for
CARDIAC IMPLANTABLE DEVICES

Workbook of Diagnostics for
CARDIAC IMPLANTABLE DEVICES

David L. Hayes, MD

James D. Ryan, RN

Siva K. Mulpuru, MD

Nora E. Olson, RN

Tracy L. Webster, RN

Yong-Mei Cha, MD

Mark J. Henrich, RN

Jon M. Meyer, RN

Michael J. Hillestad, RN

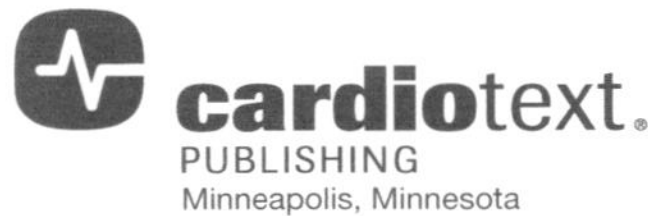

cardiotext.
PUBLISHING
Minneapolis, Minnesota

Cardiotext Publishing, LLC
750 2nd St NE Suite 102
Hopkins, MN 55343
USA

www.cardiotextpublishing.com

Any updates to this book may be found at:
www.cardiotextpublishing.com/electrophysiology-heart-rhythm-mgmt/workbook-of-diagnostics

Comments, inquiries, and requests for bulk sales can be directed to the publisher at:
info@cardiotextpublishing.com

Library of Congress Control Number: 2019956414

ISBN: 978-1-942909-38-5

eISBN: 978-1-942909-45-3

6 5 4 3

Contents

Contributors. vii

Preface ix

Abbreviations xi

Case Studies

  1. Variation in Paced QRS Morphology 1

  2. Ventricular Undersensing in a Dual-Chamber Pacemaker 3

  3. Atrial Pacing with a Competing Junctional Rhythm 5

  4. Loss of AV Synchrony 9

  5. Postventricular Atrial Refractory Period (PVARP) Function. 11

  6. Atrial Loss of Capture 13

  7. Loss of Capture and Pseudofusion. 17

  8. Loss of RV and LV Capture 21

  9. Atrial Undersensing 23

10. Functional Atrial Undersensing 25

11. Undersensing of Atrial Arrhythmia 27

12. Ventricular Safety Pacing 29

13. DDI Pacing Mode. 33

14. Functional Ventricular Undersensing. 35

15. Atrial Sensed Events in Refractory Period 37

16. Pseudo-Wenckebach Upper Rate Behavior (Medtronic). 41

17. Pseudo-Wenckebach Upper Rate Behavior (Boston Scientific). 43

18. Pseudo-Wenckebach Upper Rate Behavior (St. Jude Medical*) 45

19. His Pacing Threshold at Implant. 47

20. Crosstalk Oversensing on Ventricular Channel with His Pace/Sense Lead in RV Port 51

21. Pseudo Undersensing in Leadless Pacemaker 53

22. Remote Alert Follow-Up. 55

23. Promoting Intrinsic Ventricular Conduction. 59

24. Atrial Preference Pacing. 61

25. Rate Drop Response 63

26. Rate Smoothing. 65

*St. Jude Medical is now Abbott.

27. Atrial Flutter Response 67

28. Atrial Tachyarrhythmia with Atrial Intervention Pacing. 69

29. Mode Switch Termination with Failure to Establish AV Synchrony. 71

30. Inappropriate Mode Switch 73

31. Loss of AV Synchrony Due to Inappropriate Mode Switch 77

32. Auto-PVARP and Inappropriate Mode Switch 81

33. Pacemaker-Mediated Tachycardia 85

34. Pacemaker-Mediated Tachycardia Intervention 89

35. Pacemaker-Mediated Tachycardia in CRT-P 91

36. Respiratory Trends and Atrial Oversensing 95

37. Signal Artifact Monitor 97

38. Ventricular Noise Reversion 101

39. Ventricular Oversensing with RV Lead Failure 105

40. Atrial Oversensing 107

41. Noise Oversensing 109

42. Electromagnetic Interference in ICD 111

43. RV Lead Failure. 113

44. RV Lead Fracture 115

45. Atrial Oversensing with Inappropriate Mode Switch and Arrhythmia Induction 117

46. Short-Long-Short-Induced Ventricular Tachycardia 119

47. Managed Ventricular Pacing Mode and Ventricular Arrhythmias 123

48. Ventricular Pacing in the Vulnerable Period Due to Blanking and Associated Arrhythmia . . .127

49. Ventricular Pacing in the Vulnerable Period During Atrial Flutter 131

50. T-Wave Oversensing 135

51. RV Lead Integrity Warning and T-Wave Oversensing Discrimination 137

52. Subcutaneous ICD Oversensing 141

53. Mode Switch During VT Detection 145

54. Single-Chamber ICD with Atrial Sensing 153

55. Medtronic Detection Zones with Fast VT via VT versus Fast VT via VF 157

56. Ventricular Tachycardia Detection and Therapy. 161

57. Ventricular Tachycardia Accelerating to Ventricular Fibrillation with Undersensing 163

58. Defibrillator Therapy Following Episode Termination 169

59. Effective CRT 173

60. CRT Pacing Diagnostics 177

61. CRT Pacing Diagnostics 181

Appendix A: Cases by Title 185

Appendix B: Cases by Manufacturer 187

Contributors

David L. Hayes, MD
Consultant, Department of Cardiovascular Medicine, Mayo Clinic, Rochester, Minnesota; Professor of Medicine, Mayo Clinic College of Medicine and Science

James D. Ryan, RN
Registered Nurse, Department of Nursing, Cardiology Division, Heart Rhythm Services, Mayo Clinic, Rochester, Minnesota

Siva K. Mulpuru, MD
Consultant, Department of Cardiovascular Medicine, Mayo Clinic, Rochester, Minnesota; Associate Professor of Medicine, Mayo Clinic College of Medicine and Science

Nora E. Olson, RN
Registered Nurse, Department of Nursing, Cardiology Division, Heart Rhythm Services, Mayo Clinic, Rochester, Minnesota

Tracy L. Webster, RN
Registered Nurse, Department of Nursing, Cardiology Division, Heart Rhythm Services, Mayo Clinic, Rochester, Minnesota

Yong-Mei Cha, MD
Consultant, Department of Cardiovascular Medicine, Mayo Clinic, Rochester, Minnesota; Professor of Medicine, Mayo Clinic College of Medicine and Science

Mark J. Henrich, RN
Registered Nurse, Department of Nursing, Cardiology Division, Heart Rhythm Services, Mayo Clinic, Rochester, Minnesota; Instructor in Nursing, Mayo Clinic College of Medicine and Science

Jon M. Meyer, RN
Registered Nurse, Department of Nursing, Cardiology Division, Heart Rhythm Services, Mayo Clinic, Rochester, Minnesota

Michael J. Hillestad, RN
Registered Nurse, Department of Nursing, Cardiology Division, Heart Rhythm Services, Mayo Clinic, Rochester, Minnesota

Preface

"The world is the true classroom. The most rewarding and important type of learning is through experience, seeing something with our own eyes."

—Jack Hanna

In order to understand cardiac implantable electronic device (CIED) management, the clinician requires a foundation of information regarding CIED purpose, design, and function, as well as experience in interpreting CIED output, i.e., electrical assessment of the system, programmed parameters, electrograms, and markers. In addition, one must be able to correlate and interpret the accompanying electrocardiographic tracing with the patient's clinical presentation.

As I've encountered students of CIED management, be they beginners in the field or more advanced students of CIED, there is always an appreciation for case studies, i.e., real-world examples of managing a specific device-related issue.

In our practice, we see opportunities every day for teaching CIED management, coming from the clinic, the bedside, and remote transmissions. These are rich examples that range from very simple and straightforward clinical management issues to more complex issues that may be related to a specific device algorithm.

The Heart Rhythm Service practice at the Mayo Clinic is supported by a talented group of RN Device Specialists who are trained "on the job." The RN Device Specialists manage the vast majority of our day-to-day CIED patient encounters. They are involved in device implantation, pre-and postoperative management, patient education, in-clinic and bedside programming, and troubleshooting, as well as initial interpretation of all remote transmissions.

This text has been prepared by six of our talented RN Device Specialists and three physicians involved in our Heart Rhythm Services. (Some cases were contributed by Dean Engle, RN, Katherine Lukkason, RN, and Francisco [Kit] Gatcheco, RN.)

We have collected examples from pacemakers, ICDs, and CRT devices, illustrating interpretation, and management of a variety of device behaviors, some with abnormal function that requires diagnosis and management approach, and others that display appropriate behavior of a specific device algorithm that may be confusing for the CIED student. We have attempted to organize the cases from basic concepts to more complex device issues.

We have adapted a successful format from friends and colleagues in France who have developed a large series of device management cases (cardiocases.com, a data bank of theoretical teaching and practical clinical training, StimuPrat Ed., FR).

Our cases follow a specific format:

- Title describing the topic of the case

- Type of device, manufacturer, and model

- Brief patient/scenario description

- Presentation of the EGM and other pertinent tracings or programmed parameters

    - Figures include numerical notations, e.g., [111], that correspond to a specific finding that is important in terms of understanding the case

    - The same notations then correlate with the explanatory text that follows

- EGM analysis that includes individual teaching points/explanations, and included within the text are corresponding numerical references, e.g., [2] correlates with [111] on the EGM

- Clinical response—a brief explanation of what management was required as a result of the issue described

We have learned a great deal as we developed and reviewed the clinical cases included in this book. Despite a detailed and sequenced review process with each case being scrutinized by multiple authors, there are no doubt cases where readers may have a difference of opinion or see some nuance or other teaching point that was included in the description. We welcome your feedback on the cases as we hope to make this a dynamic process and continue to add cases to our collections. We also welcome any cases you may wish to share for inclusion in a subsequent edition that would be credited appropriately. Please contact us at cases@cardiotextpublishing.com.

—David L. Hayes, MD, and the contributors

Abbreviations

AF   atrial fibrillation
AFR   Atrial Flutter Response [Boston Scientific device setting]
AMS   automatic mode switch
APP   Atrial Preference Pacing [Medtronic device setting]
ARVC   arrhythmogenic right ventricular cardiomyopathy
AS   atrial sensed
AT   atrial tachycardia
ATP   antitachycardia pacing
ATR   atrial tachycardia rate
AV   atrioventricular
AVD   atrioventricular delay

BiV   biventricular
bpm   beats per minute

CABG   coronary artery bypass grafting
CHF   congestive heart failure
CI   confidence interval
CIED   cardiac implantable electronic device
CLS   closed-loop stimulation
CRT   cardiac resynchronization therapy
CRT-D   cardiac resynchronization therapy + defibrillator
CRT-P   cardiac resynchronization therapy + pacemaker
CT   computed tomography

ECG   electrocardiogram
ED   emergency department
EF   ejection fraction
EGM   electrogram
EMI   electromagnetic interference
ERP   effective refractory period

FARI   filtered atrial rate interval
FFRW   far-field R wave

ICD	implantable cardioverter-defibrillator
J	joule

L	liter
LV	left ventricle; left ventricular
LVAD	left ventricular assist device
LVEF	left ventricular ejection fraction
LVRP	left ventricular refractory period

MI	myocardial infarction
MRI	magnetic resonance imaging
MTR	maximum tracking rate
MV	minute ventilation

NC	no capture
NCAP	noncompetitive atrial pacing
NSVT	nonsustained ventricular tachycardia
NYHA	New York Heart Association

OR	odds ratio

PAC	premature atrial complex
PAVBP	postatrial ventricular blanking period
PMT	pacemaker-mediated tachycardia
PVAB	postventricular atrial blanking
PVABP	postventricular atrial blanking period
PVARP	postventricular atrial refractory period
PVC	premature ventricular complex

RV	right ventricular

SAM	signal artifact monitor
SVC	superior vena cava

TARP	total atrial refractory period
TIM	transthoracic impedance measurements

VA	ventriculoatrial
VF	ventricular fibrillation
VIP	ventricular intrinsic preference
VS	ventricular sensed
VT	ventricular tachycardia

1 | Variation in Paced QRS Morphology

DEVICE: St. Jude Medical* Accent DR 2110 DC PM

PATIENT: An 82-year-old patient with a history of chronic atrial fibrillation receives a single-chamber pacemaker for symptomatic bradycardia. At a routine in-clinic follow-up, the EGM tracing (**Figure 1**) was obtained.

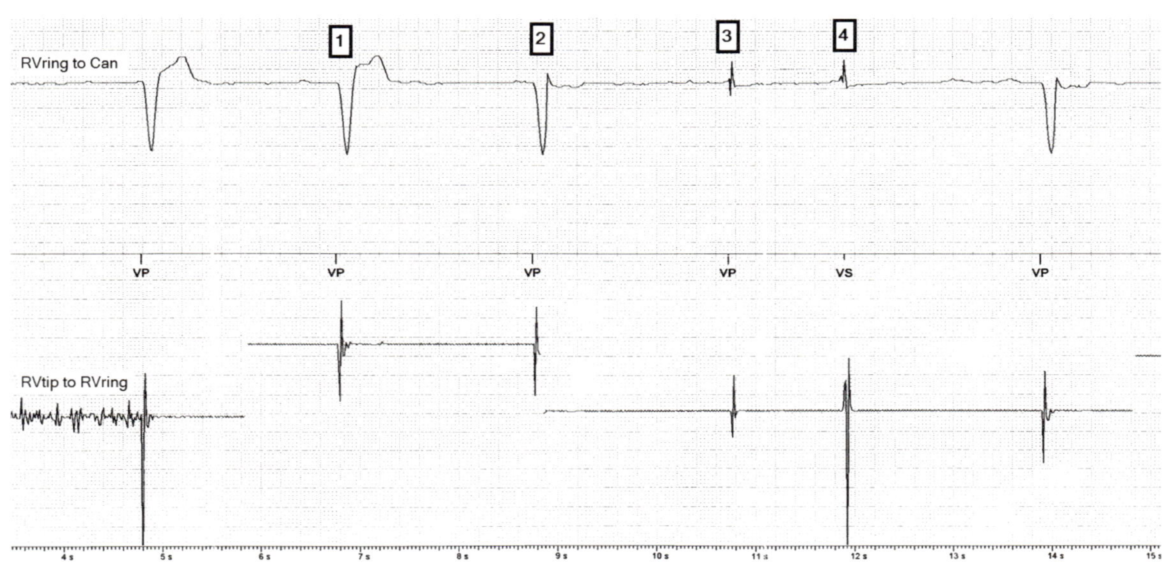

Figure 1.

ANALYSIS

1. The first two QRS complexes share the same wide QRS morphology and represent a true ventricular paced beat.

2. The third complex is not the same as the first two QRS complexes, i.e., the QRS is narrower, but significantly different than the single ventricular sensed beat seen later in the tracing [4]. This represents a ventricular fusion beat (fusion of paced and conducted wavefronts).

---

*St. Jude Medical is now Abbott.

3. The QRS complex labeled [3] appears identical to the QRS complex that follows [4] but is a paced ventricular beat as evidenced by the "marker" below, and indeed a pacing artifact can be seen on the narrow QRS complex. This represents a pseudofusion ventricular beat. Pseudofusion occurs when the local ventricular activation near the pacing lead occurs late in the inscribed QRS. The timing cycle expires, resulting in ventricular pacing. However, the ventricular pacing may capture the local myocardium and does not contribute much to change the QRS complex and is therefore identified as a pseudofusion beat. It takes about 20% of the ventricular myocardial activation from a wavefront to appreciate fusion on surface ECG.

4. This QRS complex is the only sensed ventricular beat in the tracing (VS) and represents a true intrinsic beat.

CLINICAL RESPONSE

This tracing represents entirely normal function. It is important to be able to recognize the difference between intrinsic and wholly paced beats from fusion and pseudofusion complexes.

2 | Ventricular Undersensing in a Dual-Chamber Pacemaker

DEVICE: Medtronic Advisa DR MRI A2DR01 DC PM

PATIENT: An 80-year-old male had a dual-chamber pacemaker implanted for intermittent, symptomatic second-degree heart block two years ago. The EGM tracing in **Figure 2a** was obtained during routine in-clinic pacemaker interrogation. Pertinent programmed parameters are shown in **Figure 2b**. What is the problem in this tracing?

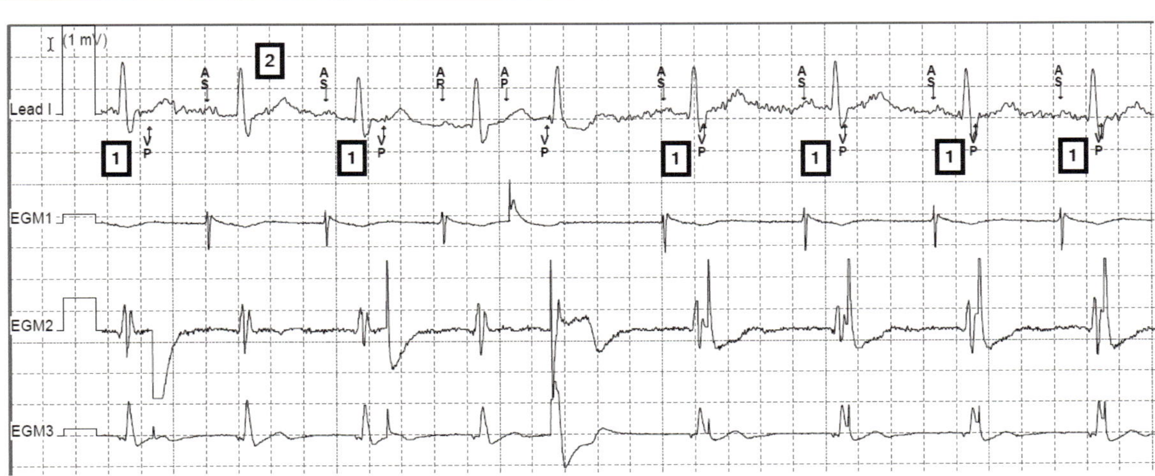

Figure 2a.

Parameter Summary

Mode	2 AAI ⟷ DDD	Lower Rate	60 bpm	Paced AV	250 ms
Mode Switch	171 bpm	Upper Track	130 bpm	Sensed AV	250 ms
		Upper Sensor	130 bpm		

Figure 2b.

ANALYSIS

1. The surface lead, lead I, shows an intrinsic QRS that is not sensed, as indicated by the lack of a VS event marker. The QRS is then followed by a VP. The ventricular lead was programmed pace/sense bipolar. Bipolar R wave measured 0.5 mV to 1.2 mV during interrogation and RV sensitivity was set to nominal bipolar value of 0.9 mV.

2. Medtronic's MVP algorithm is in effect, which changed pacing mode to DDDR with programmed A-V delay of 250 ms. Please refer to Medtronic's manual for complete algorithm functionality.

The patient denied any symptoms that could be related to heart rate or rhythm. The R wave had shown slight, gradual decrease in amplitude since implant. The RV impedance and threshold have appeared to remained stable since implant. The R-wave unipolar measured 5.0 mV. RV thresholds both unipolar and bipolar were the same and no extracardiac stimulation noted when pacing unipolar at max outputs. Provocative maneuvers to elicit oversensing of myopotentials were seen at RV sensitivity of 2.0 mV, but not at the nominal unipolar sensitivity of 2.8 mV. Due to this, and the patient's lack of pacemaker dependency, the RV was left as pace bipolar and sensing was changed to unipolar with a sensitivity of 2.8 mV. The patient will require close follow-up via CareLink remote transmission or clinic checks to identify future lead issues.

Atrial and ventricular leads are programmed to bipolar pace/sense. The measured R wave ranged from 0.5 mV to 1.2 mV bipolar and the device was programmed with RV sensitivity at the nominal bipolar value of 0.9 mV. This resulted in frequent undersensing and inappropriate or "overpacing" of the RV as seen above. Other lead trends were stable.

Atrial Pacing with a Competing Junctional Rhythm

DEVICE: Medtronic Adapta ADDR01 DC PM

PATIENT: A 75-year-old male with a history of paroxysmal atrial fibrillation had a dual-chamber pacemaker implanted for junctional bradycardia following mitral valve replacement and a maze procedure. One year later, after developing significant tricuspid valve regurgitation, the RV lead was explanted and the device was programmed to AAI mode at 80 bpm with an atrial amplitude of 5.0 V with a pulse width of 0.4 ms. The pacemaker nurse specialist was called to interrogate the device due to concerns for loss of atrial capture as evidenced by a change in rhythm on the monitor and a heart rate frequently below the programmed lower rate limit of 80 bpm. The bedside nurse noted that the monitor showed irregular conduction of atrial pacing impulses, which represented a change from what was previously seen on the monitor when atrial pacing at 80 bpm with 1:1 conduction was consistently seen. Presenting rhythm (**Figure 3a**), underlying rhythm (**Figure 3b**), atrial threshold testing (**Figure 3c**), and atrial pacing at 100 bpm (**Figure 3d**) are shown.

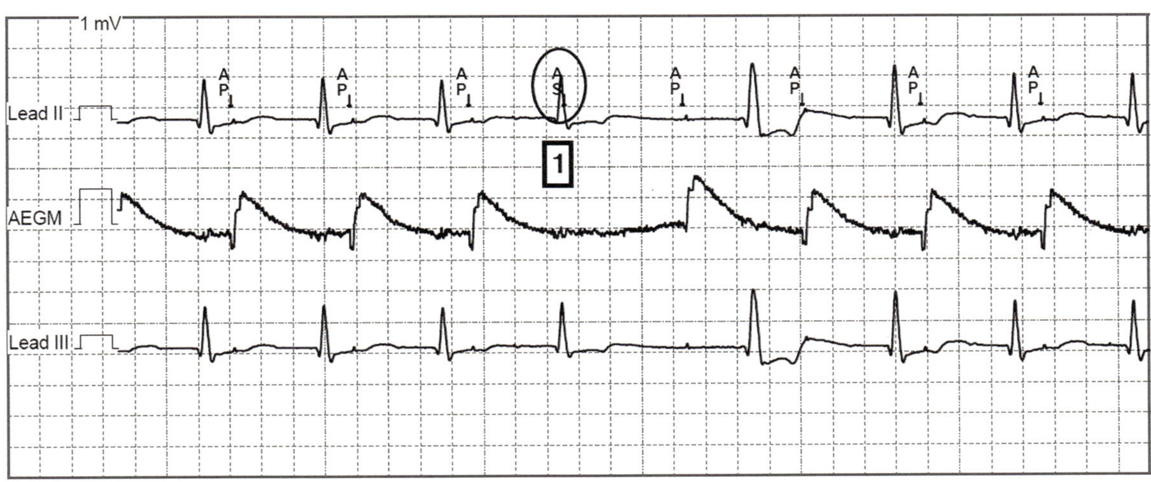

Figure 3a.

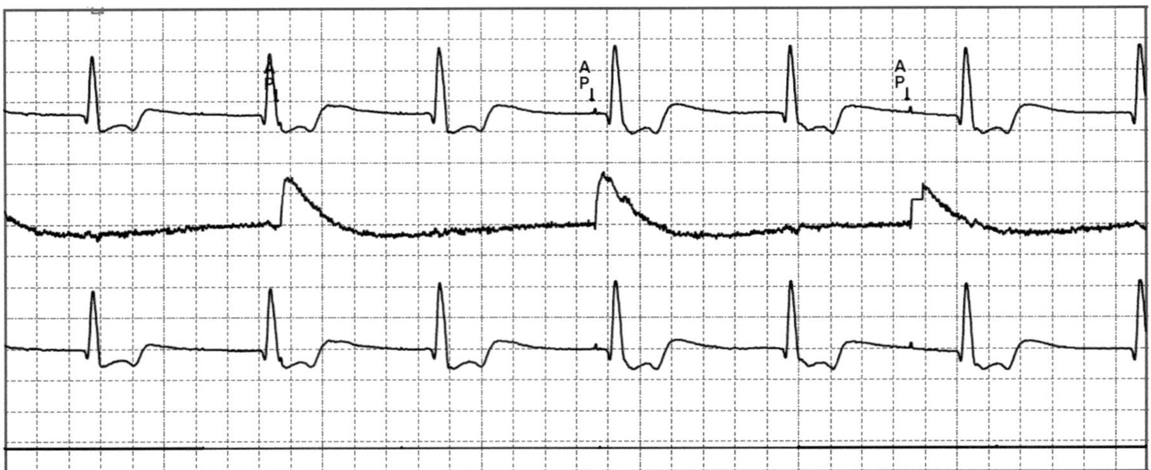

Figure 3b.

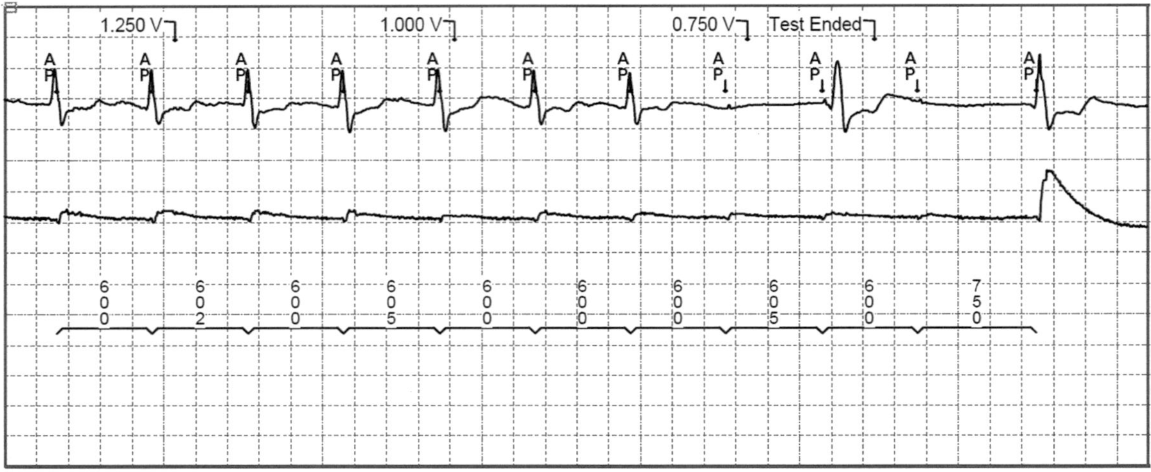

Figure 3c.

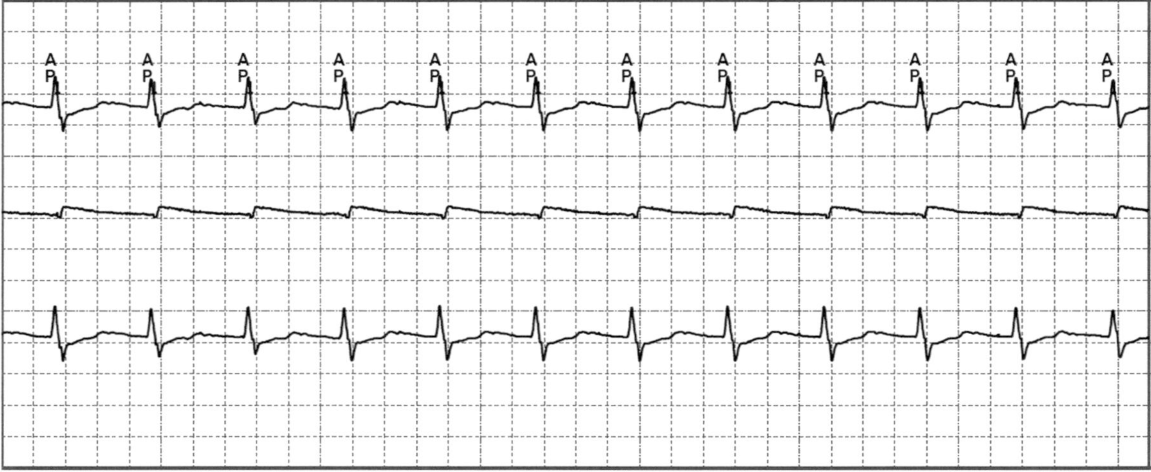

Figure 3d.

ANALYSIS

1. In Figure 3a, the presenting EGM shows atrial pacing at 80 bpm with a variable ventricular rate ranging from 50 to 80 bpm. This variable rate occurs when the far-field R wave (FFRW), sensed by the atrial lead, inhibits atrial pacing [1]. Inspecting the tracing in a vertical fashion demonstrates that the QRS complex is noted on the atrial EGM as a sensed atrial (AS) event. After pacing stimulus, polarization is seen on the sensing electrode, and it decays with time. When the decay point is more than the set sensitivity or when far-field signals exceed the threshold, atrial events are declared and pacing is withheld.

2. In Figure 3b, device was programmed AAI at 30 bpm for a P-wave amplitude test revealing no sensed P waves, atrial pacing at 30 bpm, and a junctional escape rhythm at a rate of 56 bpm.

3. To confirm atrial capture, an atrial threshold test was conducted with AAI pacing at 100 bpm, revealing a threshold of 1.0 V at 0.4 ms (see Figure 3c).

4. Programming the device AAI at 100 bpm showed 1:1 conduction with an AP interval of 600 ms, as seen in Figure 3d. However, given the short AP interval, pacing at this rate or higher is likely to produce occasional dropped beats and potential activity intolerance for the patient. The FFRW oversensing seen in Figure 3a can occur at any rate and will likely produce the irregular ventricular rate seen by the bedside nurse.

CLINICAL RESPONSE

In an attempt to reduce FFRW oversensing, the atrial sensitivity was reduced from 0.18 mV to 0.25 mV. The atrial output was adjusted based on the threshold testing. The patient was discharged from the hospital with a 30-day monitor to determine the need for ventricular pacing and a potential upgrade to a biventricular (BiV) device.

4 | Loss of AV Synchrony

DEVICE: Medtronic Evera XT DR DDBB1D4 DC ICD

PATIENT: A 39-year-old patient with a history of dilated cardiomyopathy and ventricular tachycardia is a heart transplant candidate with an ejection fraction of 18%, and a dual-chamber ICD has been implanted for primary prevention due to severe LV dysfunction. Patient complains of an "odd feeling" when relaxing before going to bed or when lying in bed before sleep. The presenting EGM from the patient's most recent routine remote transmission is shown in **Figure 4**. The patient's atrial lead is known to have persistent failure to capture; atrial sensing is appropriate.

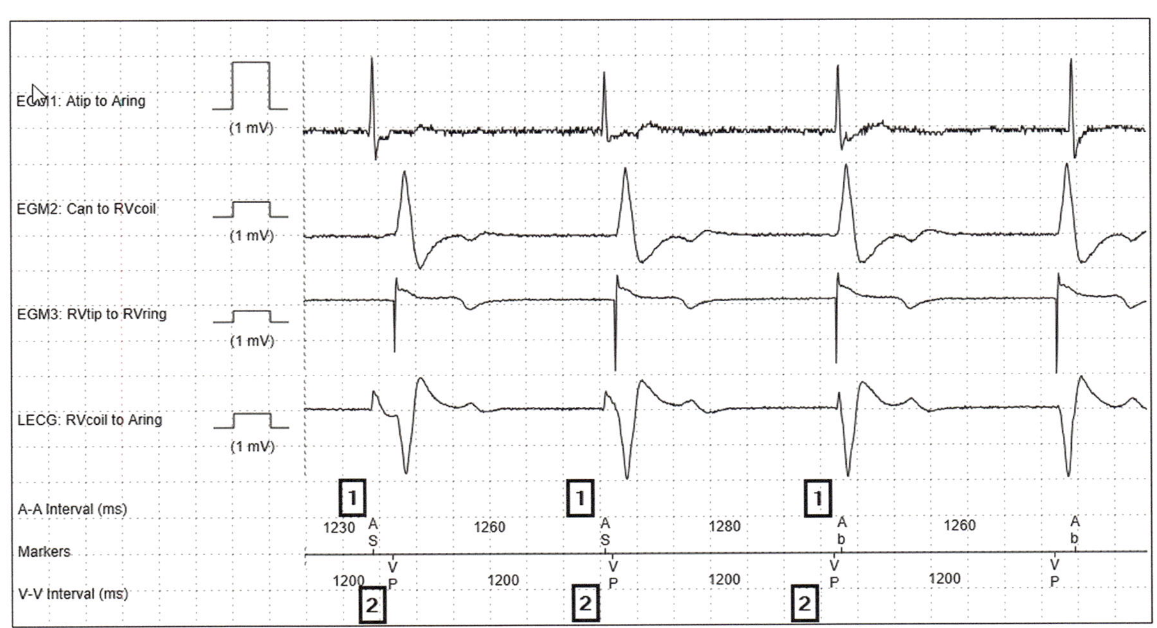

Figure 4.

ANALYSIS

1. The atrial sensed events [1] are not synchronized with the ventricular paced events [2].

2. The pacing mode is currently programmed VVI at 50 bpm. The device is functioning as programmed with ventricular pacing at 50 bpm (1200 ms). The patient's intrinsic atrial rate [1] is slower at approximately 47 bpm. This results in loss of AV synchrony. The patient is experiencing pacemaker syndrome from the loss of AV synchrony.

The single-chamber pacing mode of VVI at 50 bpm was chosen due to the atrial lead malfunction, which caused the failure to capture. This was acceptable while the patient's clinical condition did not warrant atrial pacing. AV synchrony could be restored by reprogramming the lower rate to 40 bpm. This type of programming is common in patients with single-chamber ICDs who do not require pacing support for bradycardia. Programming a different nighttime rate or turning rate hysteresis on are other potential options. Unfortunately, this leaves the patient at risk for decompensation and worsening heart failure. As a result, atrial lead revision was advised.

5 | Postventricular Atrial Refractory Period (PVARP) Function

DEVICE: Medtronic Azure XT DR MRI W1DR01 DC PM

PATIENT: A 30-year-old patient with paroxysmal atrial fibrillation and AV conduction disorder received a dual-chamber pacemaker due to pauses resulting from flecainide administration. The presenting EGM from routine remote follow-up is shown in **Figure 5a**. Does this EGM represent appropriate device function? (Programmed parameters are shown in **Figure 5b**.)

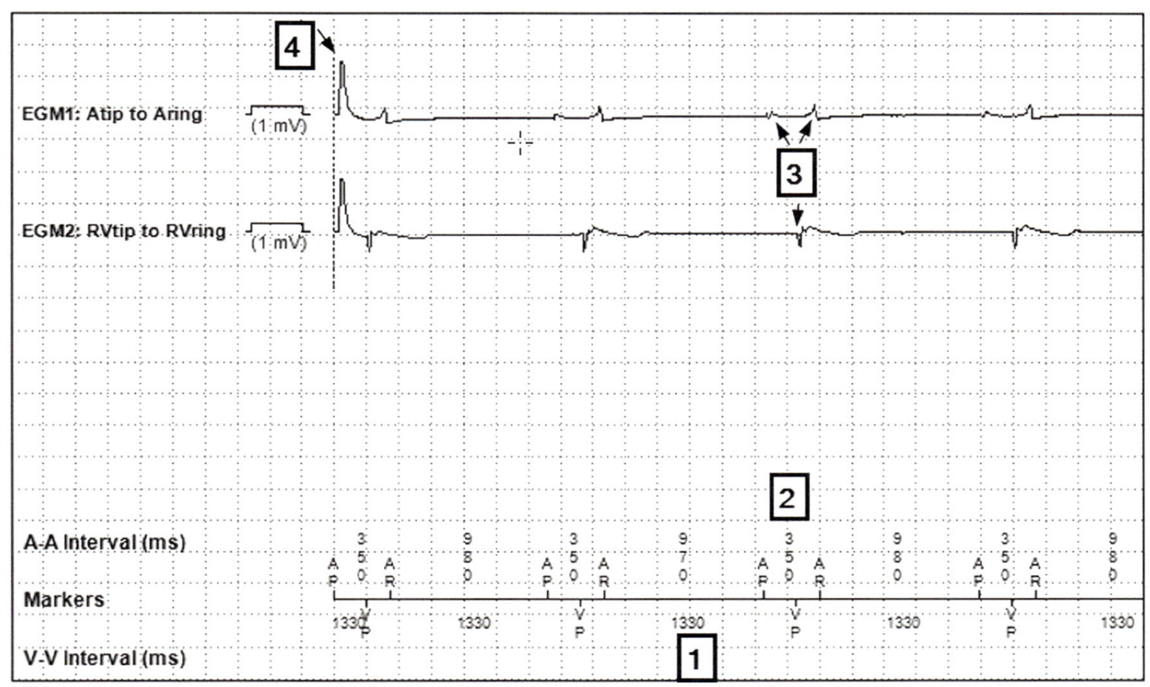

Figure 5a.

Pacing Summary

Mode		Rates		AV Intervals	
Mode	DDD	Lower	45 bpm	Paced AV	200 ms
Mode Switch	200 bpm	Upper Track	140 bpm	Sensed AV	180 ms
		Upper Sensor	130 bpm		

Refractory/Blanking

PVARP	250 ms
PVAB Interval	130 ms

Figure 5b.

ANALYSIS

1. At first glance, the 1330 ms ventricular pacing interval [1] seems unusual, but this is consistent with the programmed lower rate of 45 bpm.
   (60,000 ms/min ÷ 45 bpm = 1330 ms)

2. The channel markers [2] show a consistent and repetitive marker channel pattern of AP–VP–AR. The atrial and ventricular electrograms (EGMs) show waveforms [3] that appear to correspond with the AP, VP, and AR markers. With no sensed events to reset the timers, the AP–VP events appear appropriate with the lower rate of 45 bpm and a programmed AV interval of 200 ms.

3. The AR marker indicates that the second atrial waveform, directly following the ventricular waveform, is falling into PVARP. PVARP is programmed at a fixed duration of 250 ms. The function of PVARP in this case is to prohibit the atrial sensing of the far-field ventricular depolarization or after potential. An alternate possibility is initial failure of atrial capture with atrial sensing of retrograde conduction falling into PVARP. This scenario may warrant further in-clinic investigation.

4. What is the significance of this initial spiked waveform on both atrial and ventricular EGMs at initiation of the EGM recording? This artifact does not correspond to any of the channel markers. Medtronic technical support confirms that this is in fact artifact associated with the initiation of the EGM recording.

CLINICAL RESPONSE

Routine in-clinic follow-up confirmed atrial capture and atrial sensing of the far-field ventricular depolarization. Lead testing revealed intrinsic P waves were 0.8 mV, with a programmed atrial sensitivity of 0.45 mV. Programming the atrial sensing channel to a less sensitive value to avoid sensing of the far-field signals and eliminating the AR sense might risk undersensing the patient's atrial fibrillation episodes. Extending postventricular atrial blanking (PVAB) may have the same effect. No programming changes were made.

6 | Atrial Loss of Capture

DEVICE: St. Jude Medical* Assurity DR 2240 DC PM

PATIENT: An 81-year-old patient was implanted with a dual-chamber pacemaker for sick sinus syndrome. The patient is hospitalized following mitral valve replacement surgery for severe mitral valve stenosis. The device nurse is called to investigate the pacemaker based on the telemetry tracing shown in **Figure 6a**. The EGM from device interrogation is shown in **Figure 6b**.

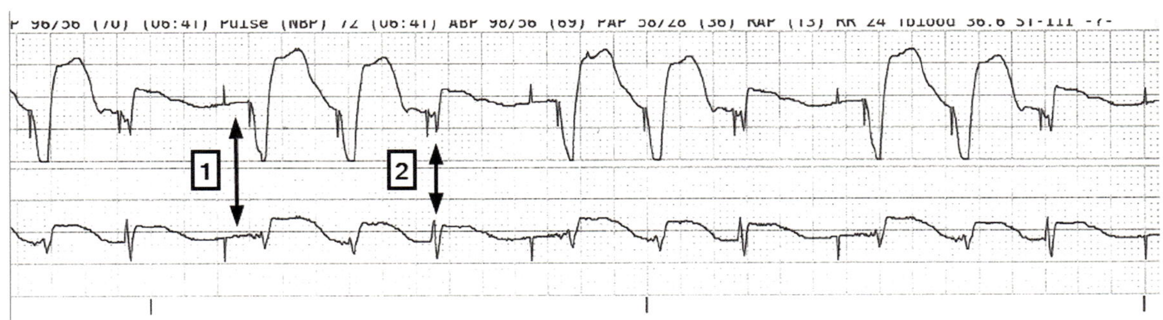

Figure 6a.

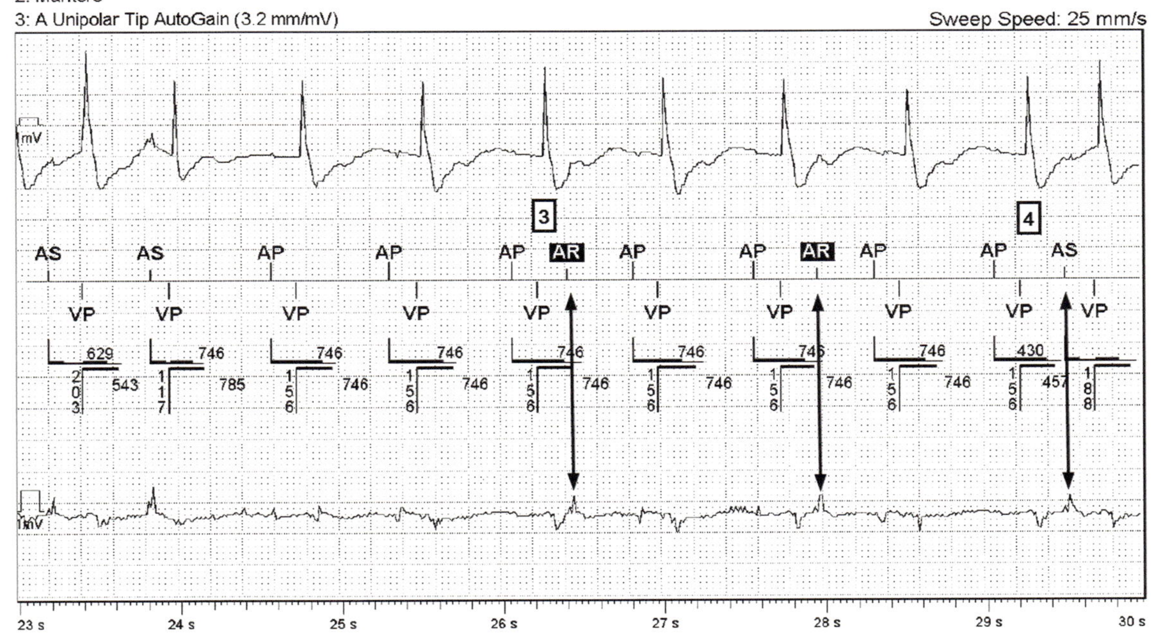

Figure 6b.

*St. Jude Medical is now Abbott.

1. Surface ECG tracings are often the first evidence of a potential device irregularity. The apparent dual paced complex at [1] appears straightforward.

2. The single paced complex at [2] results in a different waveform. Initial analysis based on the ECG strip alone suggests several possibilities, including ventricular fusion or maybe ventricular loss of capture. It is difficult to draw conclusions based solely on ECG tracings from telemetry; they can be misleading and almost always warrant further investigation, including device interrogation and testing. There is often a temptation to assume the underlying cause is benign and draw the conclusion "normal device function." Resist this temptation.

Basic Operation			
Mode	DDD		
V. Triggering	Off		
Magnet Response	Battery Test		
V. Noise Reversion Mode	VOO		
Sensor	Passive		
Threshold (Measured Avg.)	Auto (+0.0) (2.0)		
Slope (Measured Auto)	Auto (+2) (7)		
Max Sensor Rate	110 bpm		
Reaction Time	Fast		
Recovery Time	Medium		

Capture & Sense	A	V
ACap® Confirm/V. AutoCapture	Off	Off
Pulse Amplitude	3.0 V	2.0 V
Pulse Width	0.4 ms	0.4 ms
AutoSense	Off	Off
Sensitivity (Safety Margin)	0.2 mV (5:1)	1.5 mV (8:1)

Delays		
Paced AV Delay	160 ms	
Sensed AV Delay	120 ms	

Rates	
Base Rate	80 bpm
Rest Rate	Off
Max Sensor Rate	110 bpm
Max Track Rate	130 bpm
Hysteresis Rate	Off
2:1 Block Rate	186 bpm

Figure 6c.

3. The device was interrogated and the presenting EGM is shown in Figure 6b. Parameters are shown in **Figure 6c**. The EGM tracing provides further evidence and takes us in a different direction. Atrial sensed events following dual-chamber pacing [AP–VP] are observed. The atrial sensed event at [3] falls into refractory denoted by AR.

4. The atrial sensed event at [4] is in the atrial alert period, AS, and is tracked and followed by VP. These "extra" atrial sensed events correlate with waveforms on the atrial EGM. These atrial sensed events could represent premature atrial complexes (PACs) or retrograde VA conduction due to loss of atrial capture. Atrial threshold testing was performed.

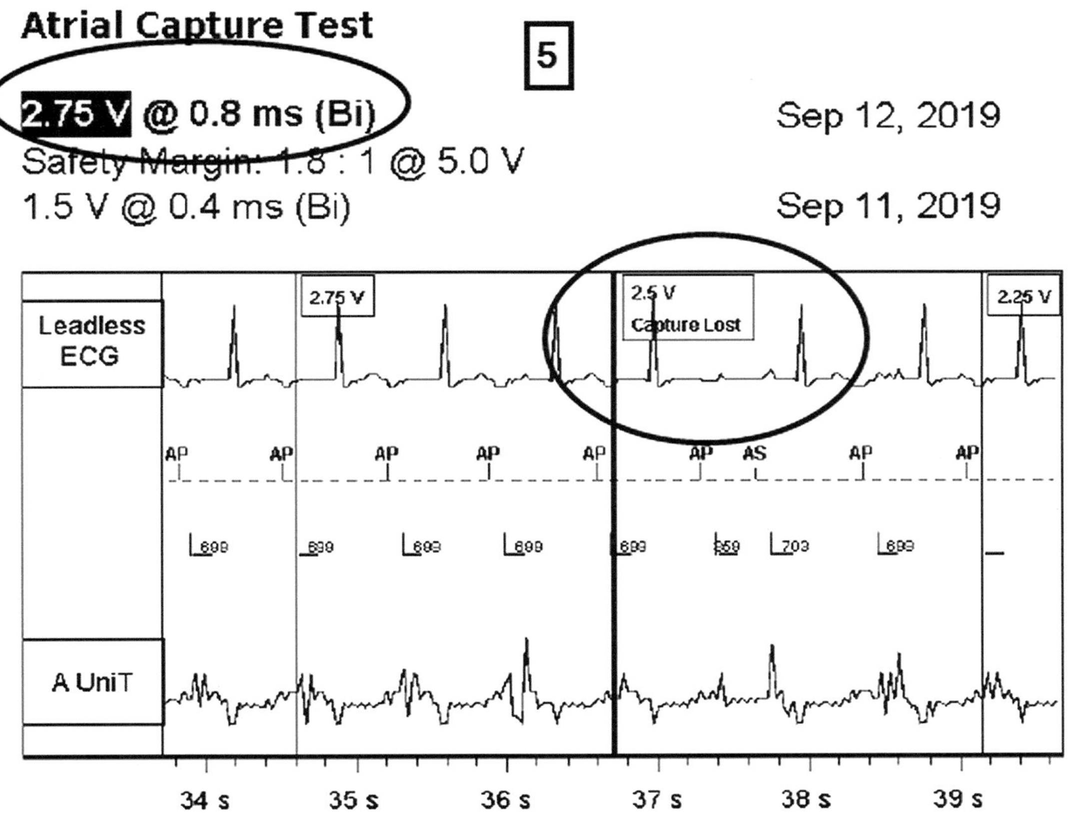

Figure 6d.

5. The atrial threshold was found to be elevated following the patient's mitral valve surgery. The threshold was 1.5 V/0.4 ms prior to surgery and measured 2.75 V/0.8 ms (**Figure 6d**) after surgery with programmed atrial output 3 V/0.4 ms. The EGM tracing most likely shows intermittent loss of atrial capture with retrograde conduction.

CLINICAL RESPONSE

The atrial output was reprogrammed to 5 V/1 ms during the patient's recovery period. There were no further irregularities observed on telemetry. It is fairly common to observe elevated atrial thresholds following cardiac surgery due to bypass cannulation of the atrium. The patient's atrial threshold subsequently returned to a level near baseline of 1.5 V/0.8 ms.

7 | Loss of Capture and Pseudofusion

DEVICE: Boston Scientific Essentio L101 DC PM

PATIENT: Patient is an 80-year-old male first implanted with a Boston Scientific Altrua dual-chamber pacemaker in 2008 for symptomatic bradycardia. Patient underwent an RV lead revision at the time of pulse generator change in 2019. The tracing in **Figure 7a** was obtained when the patient still had the original device and the original RV lead. The tracings in **Figures 7b** and **7c** are from an alert-initiated remote transmission following pulse generator change and RV lead revision.

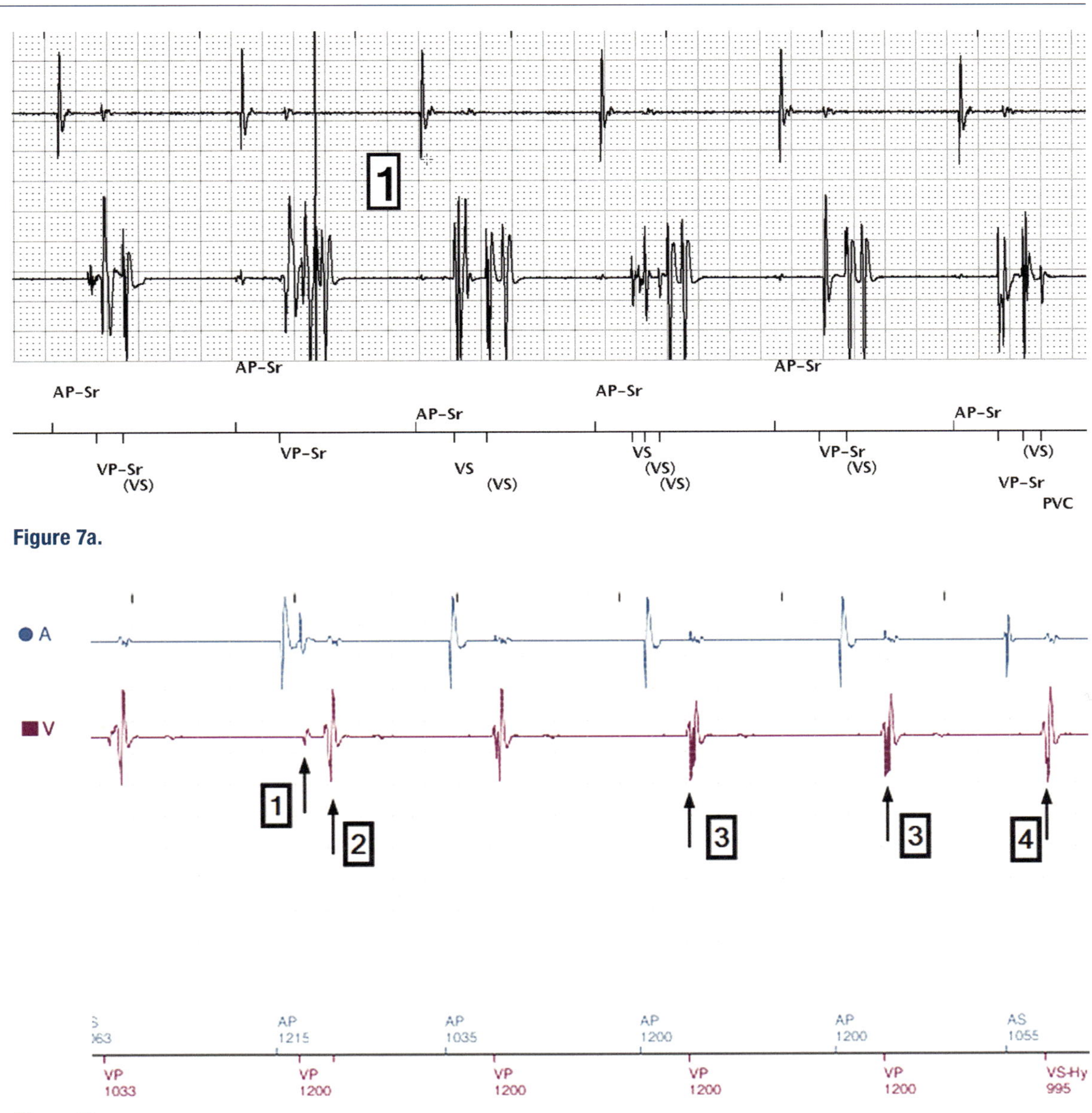

Figure 7a.

Figure 7b.

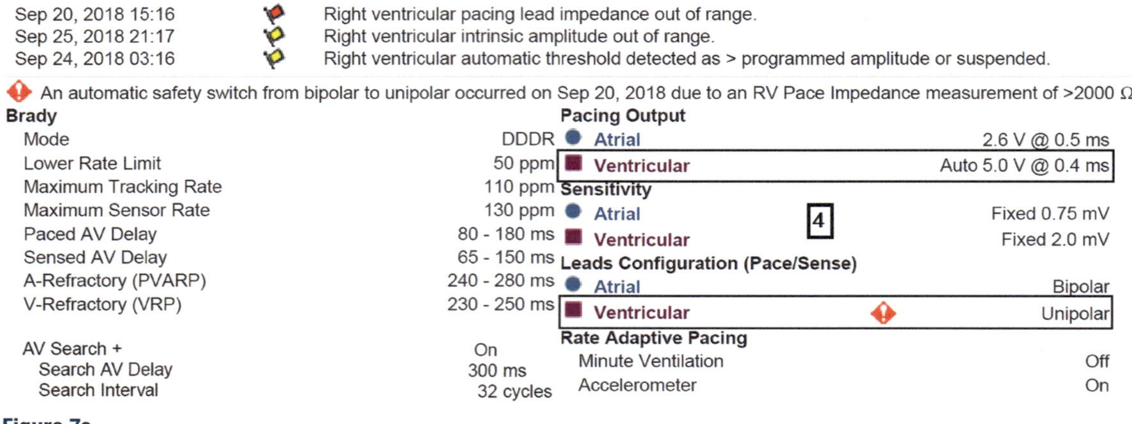

Figure 7c.

ANALYSIS

1. The tracing in Figure 7a from original device shows RV lead noise as evidenced by V-sensed markers occurring at nonphysiological intervals as short as 100 ms or less. Noise is more frequently seen after pacing or defibrillation shocks in patients with lead fracture.

2. The tracing in Figure 7b, obtained from the alert-initiated remote transmission following RV lead replacement and pulse generator change, shows loss of RV capture, apparent when the RV pacing impulse [1] is followed by a nearly 200 ms delay before the QRS complex is seen on the ventricular EGM [2]. Device assumes non-capture or high threshold when there is absence of evoked response.

3. The same tracing in Figure 7b shows pseudofusion evidenced by the RV pacing impulse [3] resulting in a QRS morphology that is identical to the V-sensed QRS morphology [4].

4. The last ventricular beat falls in the AV alert window and is sensed appropriately. The alert-initiated remote transmission was sent for polarity switch and high RV threshold as seen in Figure 7c.

Following the alert transmission, the patient was seen in the clinic. It was noted that he required essentially no ventricular pacing and therefore would realize minimal if any benefit that would warrant another RV lead revision. Atrial pacing at incremental rates was performed to verify adequacy of AV conduction. When the device was programmed to pace in AAI mode at 110 bpm, the patient had consistent 1:1 conduction. When paced at 120 bpm, there was occasional loss of AV conduction. The device was programmed to the settings seen in **Figure 7d**.

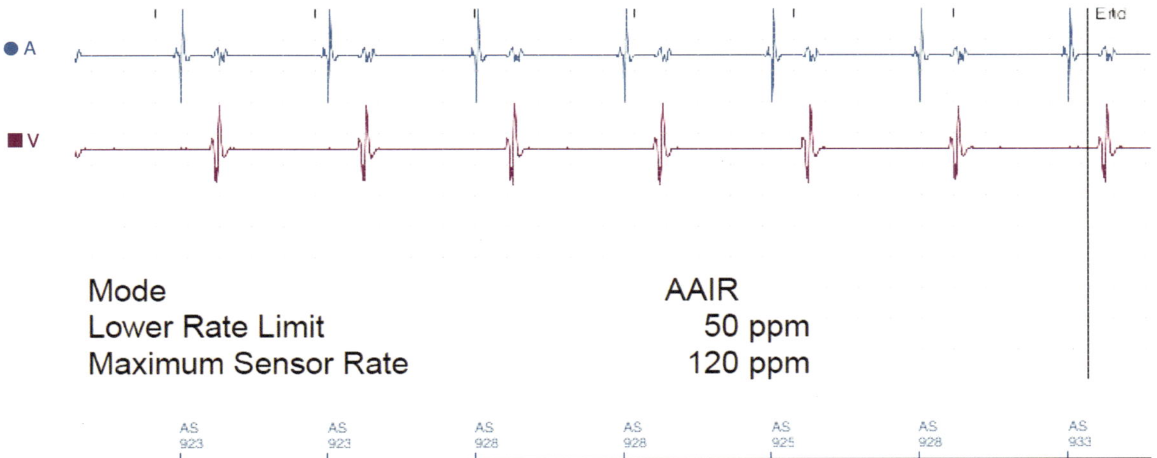

Figure 7d.

8 | Loss of RV and LV Capture

DEVICE: Medtronic Percepta Quad W4TR01 CRT-P

PATIENT: A 69-year-old patient status post aortic valve replacement due to infective cardio-myopathy underwent cardiac resynchronization therapy-pacemaker (CRT-P) device implant after developing complete heart block postoperatively. The patient was assessed four days after implant on an inpatient rehabilitative unit after complaints of "blackouts".

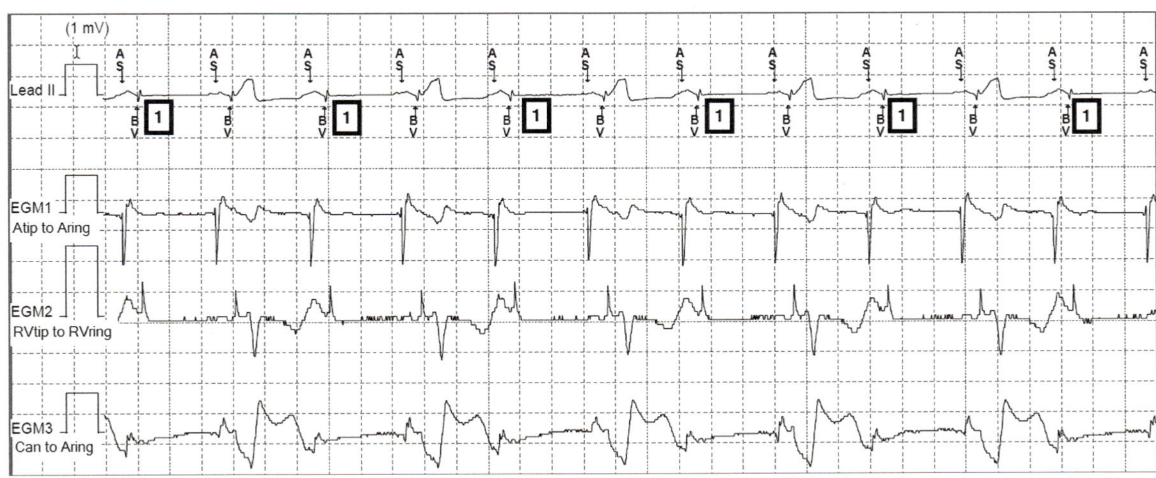

Figure 8a.

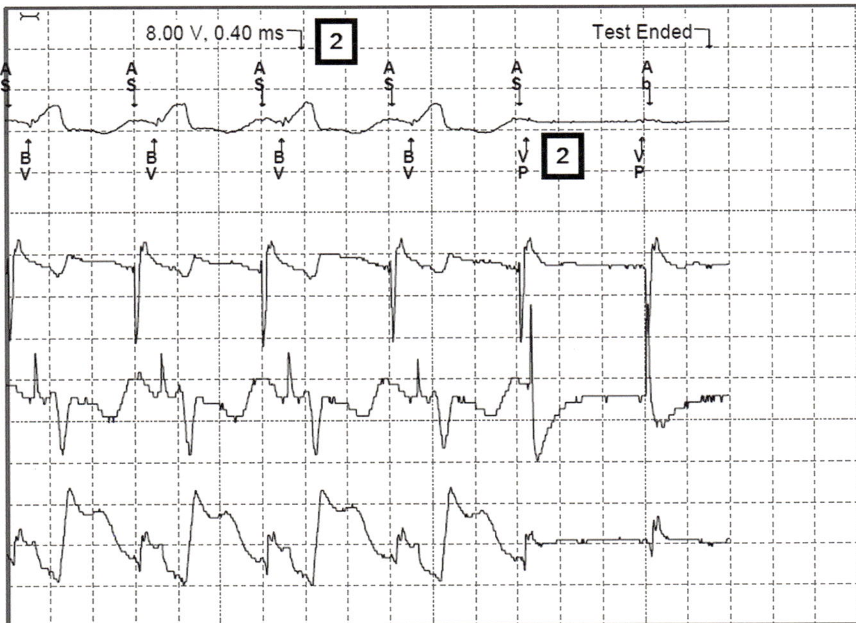

Figure 8b.

ANALYSIS

1. The presenting EGM in **Figure 8a** shows only ventricular capture with every other ventricular pacing artifact as a QRS complex only follows every other BV pace marker [1]. (Multiple simultaneous tracings are provided in the EGM which allows comparison between the tracings, i.e., vertical comparison, to more easily appreciate the alternating loss of capture.)

2. RV threshold test (**Figure 8b**) starts at 8 V/0.4 ms and did not produce any ventricular capture with the first VP (RV only pacing) marker [2]. The RV amplitude at time of this interrogation had been programmed to 3.5 V/0.4 ms causing the complete lack of RV capture. The QRS complex that is seen on the presenting EGM is the result of LV lead capture, but only with every other pacing impulse. The LV threshold was found to be 4 V/0.4 ms, the same as the currently programmed LV amplitude, resulting in the occasional loss of LV capture given the lack of any "cushion" between threshold and programmed output.

CLINICAL RESPONSE

LV amplitude was set to the max output of 8 V/1 ms to ensure LV capture and the patient underwent immediate RV lead revision. Even though thresholds were suboptimal on the LV lead, many positions had been tried at the time of the initial LV lead placement and it was not felt that lower thresholds could be achieved. Future testing of LV pacing configurations may also be performed to identify a better LV threshold.

9 | Atrial Undersensing

DEVICE: Boston Scientific Ingenio K173 DC PM

PATIENT: A 62-year-old patient had a pacemaker implanted for sinus node dysfunction and paroxysmal atrial arrhythmias. He is also status post AV node ablation and is considered pacemaker dependent. A routine quarterly remote transmission is shown below. What is demonstrated on the EGM from remote transmission shown in **Figure 9a**?

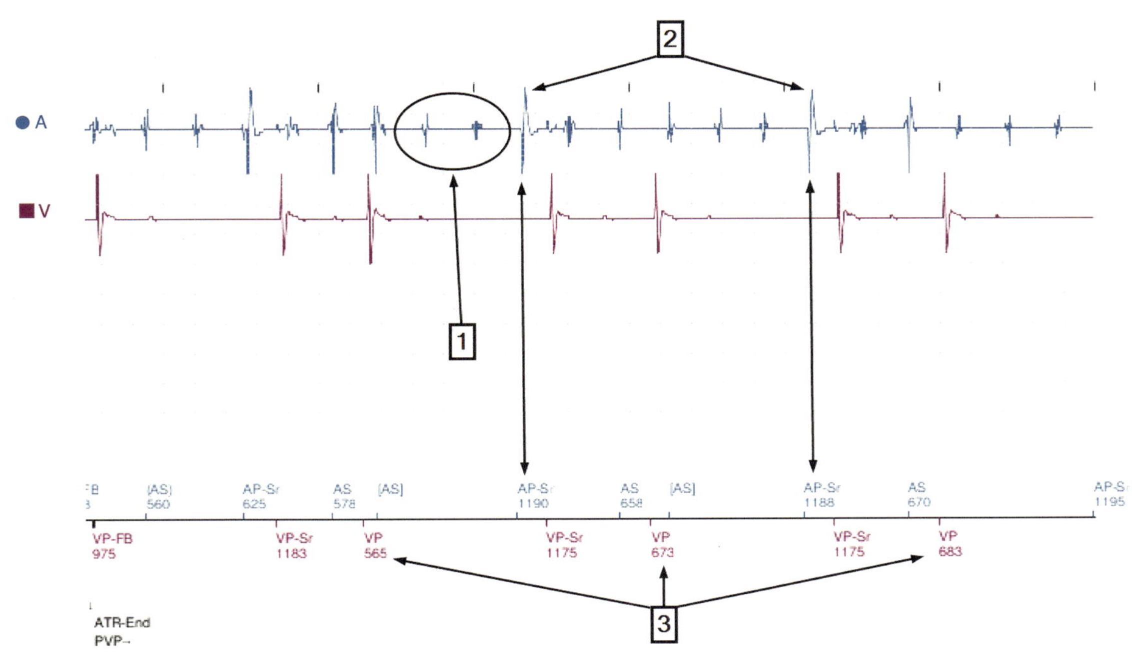

Figure 9a.

Settings

Settings		Output	
Mode	DDDR	**Output**	
RYTHMIQ™	Off	●A	4.0 V @ 0.9 ms
Lower Rate Limit	50 ppm	■V	2.5 V @ 0.4 ms
Maximum Tracking Rate	130 ppm	**Sensitivity**	
Maximum Sensor Rate	130 ppm	●A	Fixed 0.5 mV
Paced AV Delay	200 - 220 ms	■V	Fixed 2.0 mV
Sensed AV Delay	180 - 200 ms	**Leads**	
A-Refractory (PVARP)	240 - 310 ms	●A	
V-Refractory (VRP)	230 - 250 ms	Pace	Bipolar
PVARP after PVC	400 ms	Sense	Bipolar
AV Search +	Off	Safety Switch	On
Blanking		■V	
A-Blank after V-Pace	125 ms	Pace	Bipolar
A-Blank after V-Sense	45 ms	Sense	Bipolar
V-Blank after A-Pace	65 ms	Safety Switch	On

Figure 9b.

1. Intermittent undersensing of true atrial flutter P waves as evidenced by the lack of recognition of these complexes [1] on the marker channel.

2. Atrial pacing is superimposed over the atrial flutter due to the intermittent undersensing [2]. Per the marker channel, the atrial paced events AP–SR (atrial paced sensor rate) are based on the atrial timer (50 bpm or 1200 ms) following the most recent atrial event sensed in the alert period, AS.

3. Ventricular paced events are following (tracking) either atrial sensed or atrial paced events based on the programmed AV delays. The device fails to switch to atrial tachycardia mode from DDDR mode due to the atrial undersensing. The device continues to follow DDDR mode with irregular ventricular pacing [3] (Figure 9a).

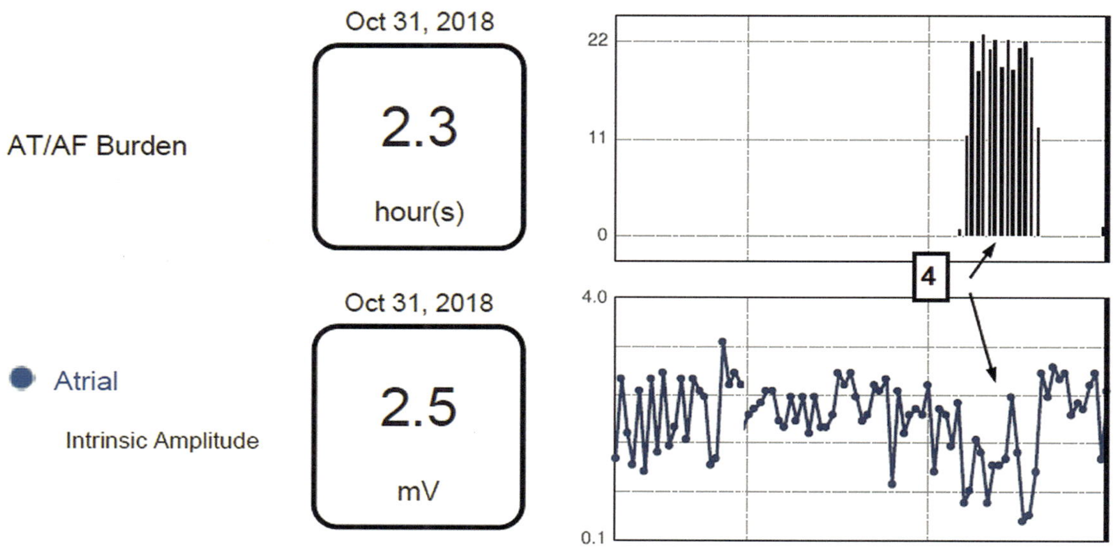

Figure 9c.

4. The atrial sensing, P wave trend [4] indicates during periods of atrial tachyarrhythmia the P wave varies to less than 0.4 mV. The current atrial sensitivity is programmed at 0.5 mV per the programmed parameters (**Figure 9b**). While the discrete P wave measurement is robust at 2.5 mV, the variations likely explain the undersensing of atrial flutter (**Figure 9c**).

CLINICAL RESPONSE

The patient was brought into the clinic for follow-up. All lead testing was within normal limits. The atrial sensitivity was increased from 0.5 mV to 0.25 mV to improve the device ability to "see" the flutter-waves. In addition, the V-Blank after V-Pace period was shortened from 150 to 100 ms to "reveal" occasional hidden atrial events, indicated by marker [AS], that are functionally blanked following ventricular pacing. These changes allowed appropriate sensing of atrial flutter with the switch to atrial tachycardia mode.

10 | Functional Atrial Undersensing

DEVICE: Boston Scientific Essentio L101 DC PM

PATIENT: An 85-year-old patient had a pacemaker implanted for sinus node dysfunction and paroxysmal atrial arrhythmias. She is also status post AV node ablation due to poor tolerance of rapid ventricular rates. The patient scheduled an in-clinic appointment due to complaints of increasing shortness of breath and feelings of "heart racing." Consider the presenting EGM recording in **Figure 10a** obtained during in-clinic pacemaker device check:

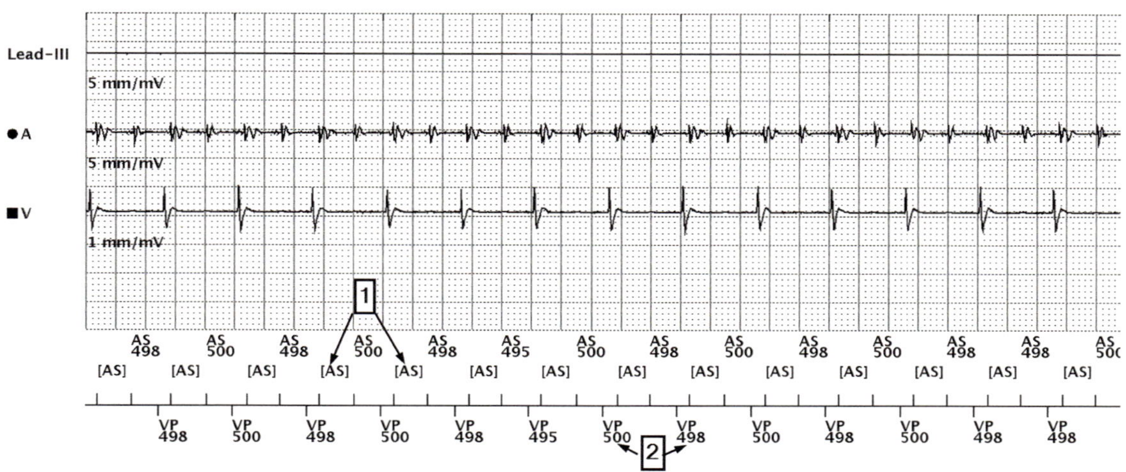

Figure 10a.

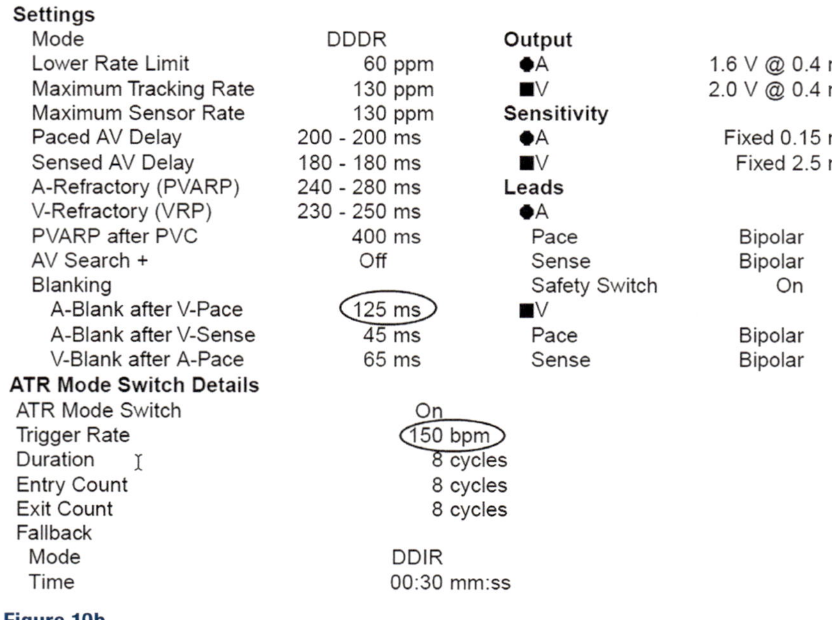

Settings

Mode	DDDR	**Output**	
Lower Rate Limit	60 ppm	●A	1.6 V @ 0.4 r
Maximum Tracking Rate	130 ppm	■V	2.0 V @ 0.4 r
Maximum Sensor Rate	130 ppm	**Sensitivity**	
Paced AV Delay	200 - 200 ms	●A	Fixed 0.15 r
Sensed AV Delay	180 - 180 ms	■V	Fixed 2.5 r
A-Refractory (PVARP)	240 - 280 ms	**Leads**	
V-Refractory (VRP)	230 - 250 ms	●A	
PVARP after PVC	400 ms	Pace	Bipolar
AV Search +	Off	Sense	Bipolar
Blanking		Safety Switch	On
A-Blank after V-Pace	125 ms	■V	
A-Blank after V-Sense	45 ms	Pace	Bipolar
V-Blank after A-Pace	65 ms	Sense	Bipolar

ATR Mode Switch Details

ATR Mode Switch	On
Trigger Rate	150 bpm
Duration	8 cycles
Entry Count	8 cycles
Exit Count	8 cycles
Fallback	
Mode	DDIR
Time	00:30 mm:ss

Figure 10b.

1. The patient appears to be in atrial flutter with an atrial rate approximately 240 bpm or an interval of 250 ms. Atrial flutter waves are noted by the alternating markers of AS and [AS]. The [AS] markers indicate atrial events in blanking [1] based on the setting A-Blank after V-Pace = 125 ms. Device settings shown in **Figure 10b**. This setting, also known as Postventricular Atrial Blanking (PVAB), ordinarily prevents atrial far-field oversensing of ventricular events. The atrial events in blanking [AS] are ignored by the device timers and are effectively "undersensed." Undersensing due to timing constraints is commonly referred to as "functional undersensing."

2. The functional atrial undersensing results in an effective atrial rate of approximately 120 bpm (500 ms). This does not meet the rate of 150 bpm at which the programmed atrial tachycardia rate (ATR) is triggered. The device follows DDDR mode with ventricular pacing [2] or tracking of AS events at 120 bpm. Patient is symptomatic due to atrial arrhythmia and ventricular pacing at a faster rate.

CLINICAL RESPONSE

All lead testing was within normal limits, including appropriate sensing of P waves. To improve functional sensing of P waves when in atrial flutter, the PVAB was shortened from 125 to 65 ms. Rate responsive AV delay was also programmed on. This also helps by effectively increasing the length of the atrial alert window. Boston Scientific devices also have AFR (atrial flutter response). It is similar to one beat mode switch and it prevents tracking of fast atrial rates. When an atrial event is sensed in the PVARP it triggers an AFR window that matches the trigger rate. Ventricular pacing is unaffected, but the atrial events in the AFR window are not tracked. Atrial pacing does not happen in AFR windows.

11 | Undersensing of Atrial Arrhythmia

DEVICE: Medtronic Claria MRI Quad DTMA1QQ CRT-D

PATIENT: A 67-year-old patient with a history of ischemic cardiomyopathy, NYHA Class II heart failure, left ventricular dysfunction (EF of 17%), and left bundle branch block (QRS of 179 ms) was implanted with a cardiac resynchronization therapy-defibrillator (CRT-D) device. The patient was in sinus rhythm at the time of CRT-D implantation. The patient called the device clinic after feeling "unwell" and sent a remote transmission with the presenting EGM shown in **Figure 11a**. Does the EGM contain any clues as to why the patient feels "unwell." Is this appropriate device function? Programmed parameters are shown in **Figure 11b**.

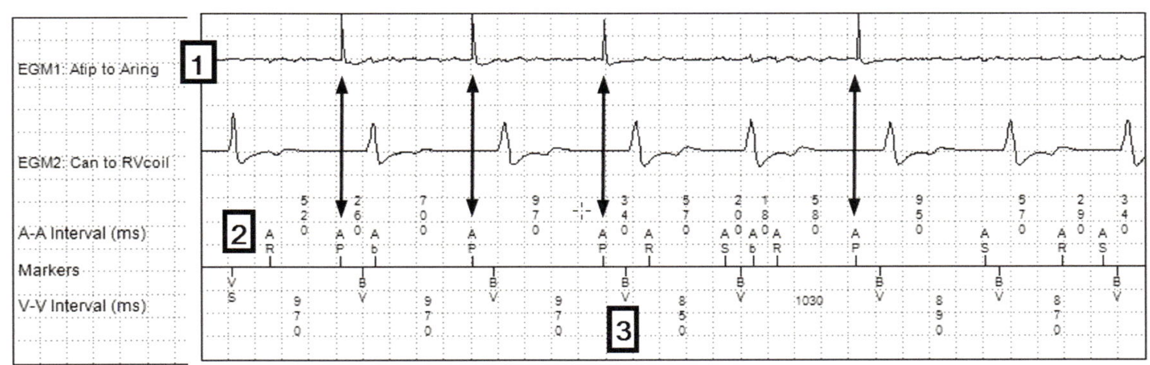

Figure 11a.

Parameter Summary

Mode	DDDR	Lower Rate	60 bpm	AdaptivCRT	Adaptive Bi-V and LV
Mode Switch	162 bpm	Upper Track	130 bpm	V. Pacing	LV->RV
		Upper Sensor	130 bpm	Paced AV	170 ms
				Sensed AV	110 ms

Detection		Rates	Therapies		
AT/AF	Monitor	>162 bpm	All Rx Off		
Pacing Details		**Atrial**	**RV**	**LV**	
Amplitude		5.00 V	3.50 V	4.50 V	
Pulse Width		1.00 ms	0.40 ms	0.40 ms	
Sensitivity		0.30 mV	0.30 mV		
Pace Polarity		Bipolar	Bipolar	LV1 to LV2	
Sense Polarity		Bipolar	Bipolar		

Figure 11b.

ANALYSIS

1. The presenting atrial EGM is suspicious for atrial arrhythmia [1]. In addition to periodic low-amplitude signals, there are pacing spikes denoted by AP markers.

2. The atrial markers [2] are irregular with both sensed and paced events. The lack of any regular sensed intervals on the atrial EGM suggests possible undersensing of atrial arrhythmia. The undersensing is intermittent, but significant enough to prevent appropriate atrial tachycardia mode switch response.

3. In this case, the biventricular (BV) pacing [3] is triggered by either tracking sensed atrial events falling in the atrial alert period, or lower-rate dual-chamber timing. Both are inappropriate. This creates an irregular ventricular paced rate. This tracing likely represents intermittent atrial undersensing of atrial fibrillation resulting in failure to mode switch.

CLINICAL RESPONSE

In-clinic follow-up assessment and 12-lead ECG confirmed new-onset atrial fibrillation. This may explain the cause of the patient's feeling "unwell." The patient was referred for atrial arrhythmia follow-up and anticoagulation assessment. Sinus P waves at implant measured 1.25 mV and atrial sensitivity by default nominal settings was programmed at 0.3 mV. Atrial fibrillatory waves measured (via remote and confirmed in clinic) 0.3 mV. The atrial sensitivity was increased from 0.3 mV to 0.15 mV. Following this programming change, appropriate atrial sensing and mode switching was achieved.

12 | Ventricular Safety Pacing

DEVICE: Medtronic Viva XT DTBA1D1 CRT-D

PATIENT: A 72-year-old patient with ischemic cardiomyopathy was implanted with a CRT-D device and also received a left ventricular assist device (LVAD). Since LVAD placement, the CRT-D has been programmed to RV pacing only with long AV delays in order to promote intrinsic conduction. The presenting EGM from a routine remote follow-up is shown in **Figure 12a**. Programmed parameters are shown in **Figure 12b**. Is safety pacing appropriate?

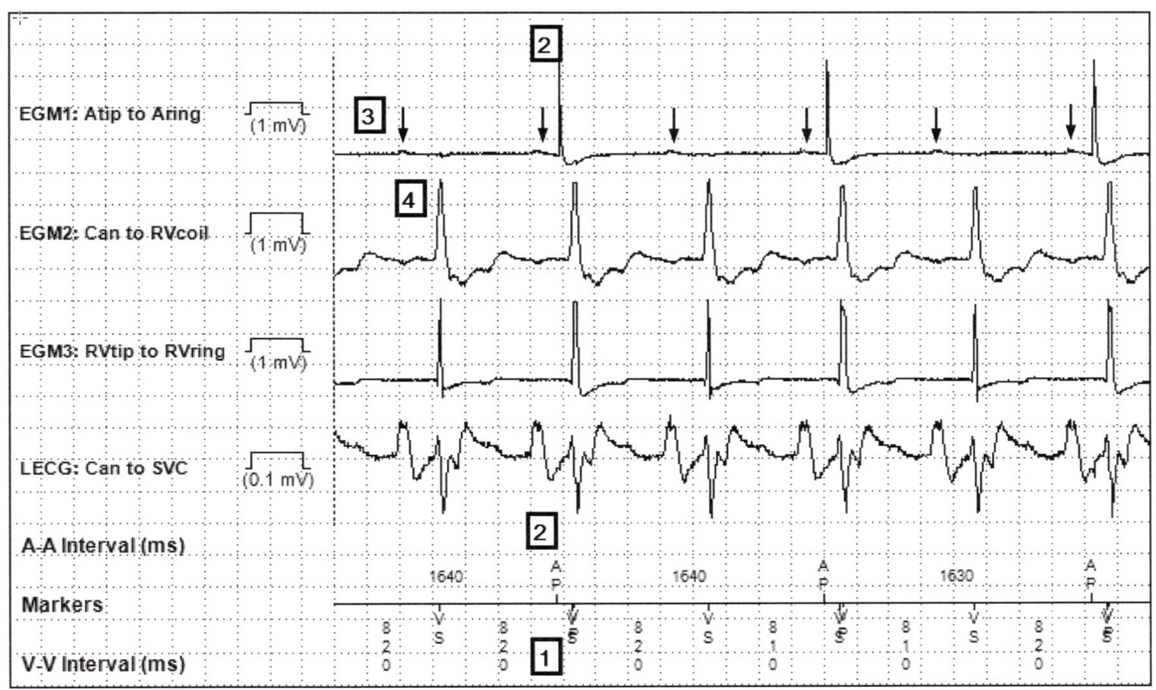

Figure 12a.

Pacing Summary

Mode		Rates		CRT	
Mode	DDDR	Lower	60 bpm	AdaptivCRT	Nonadaptive CRT
Mode Switch	171 bpm	Upper Track	120 bpm	V. Pacing	RV
		Upper Sensor	120 bpm	Paced AV	280 ms
				Sensed AV	260 ms
Sensitivity		0.30 mV	0.30 mV		
Pace Polarity		Bipolar	Bipolar		
Sense Polarity		Bipolar	Bipolar		

Figure 12b.

1. The safety pacing feature is designed to protect the patient from inhibition of ventricular pacing due to crosstalk. Crosstalk occurs when the atrial pacing impulse is sensed on the ventricular channel and inhibits ventricular pacing. When safety pacing is programmed on, the device monitors for ventricular sensed events that occur within 110 ms of an atrial paced event, also known as the "crosstalk-sensing window." This is considered a nonphysiologic AV interval or safety pace interval. When the 110 ms crosstalk sensing window expires, the device delivers a backup ventricular pacing pulse. This is indicated by the overlapping VSVP markers that are nearly coincident and the shortened AV interval [1].

2. In this case, the odd timing of the AP markers [2] and atrial EGM waveforms [3] are anomalous. The lower rate is programmed at 60 bpm (1000 ms) with a paced AV interval of 280 ms and sensed AV interval of 260 ms.

3. Closer inspection of the atrial EGM suggests undersensing of atrial events [3] that appear to consistently conduct intrinsically with the subsequent VS events [4]. (Note that the P waves that are consistently occurring [3] lack any "marker" designation, which is an indication they are not sensed by the device. (*Remember to pay as much attention to what the device doesn't label as one does to what the device does label.*)

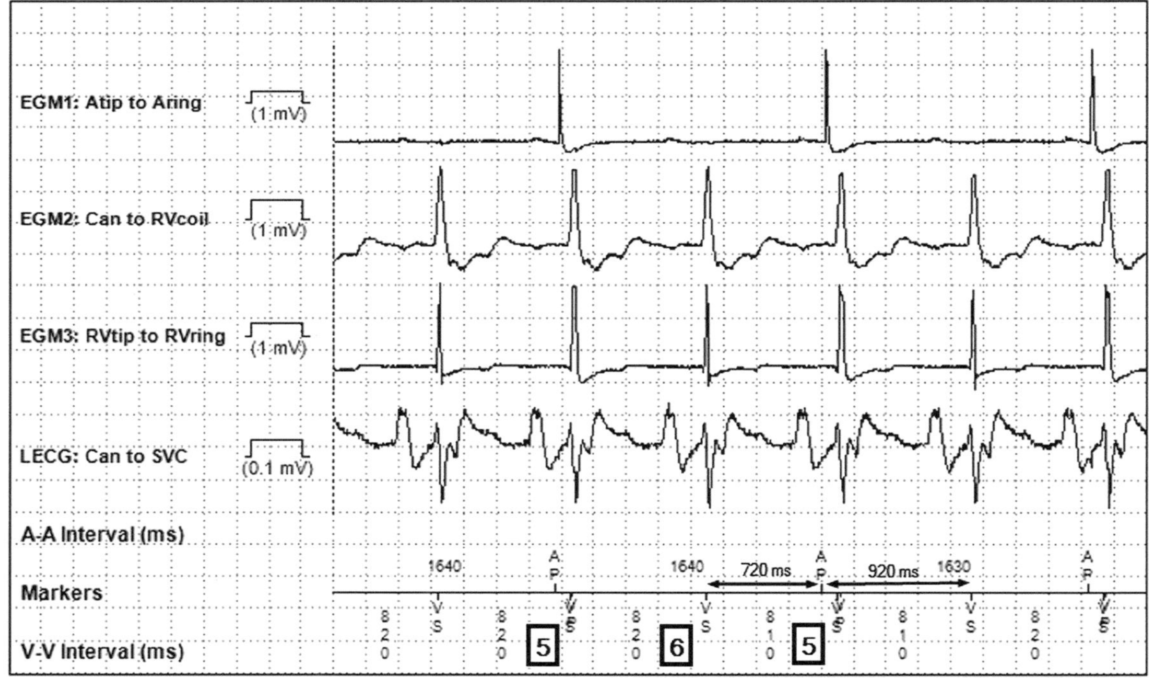

Figure 12c.

4. Given the atrial undersensing, why do we observe APVP [5] alternating with VS events [6] as shown in **Figure 12c**? The device is employing both A-to-A timing and V-to-A timing intervals. The VA interval is defined by parameters as lower rate of 1000 ms minus the PAV setting of 280 ms = 720 ms. The VS [6] with no atrial marker starts a VA timer resulting in the atrial pace 720 ms later. The APVP [5] starts an AA timer interval using the lower rate of 1000 ms. The patient's intrinsic rhythm occurs at 920 ms, which is before the scheduled atrial pace at 1000 ms, thus resetting the timer and starting the next VA interval timer of 720 ms. The scenario repeats itself, alternating between the two timing schemes.

CLINICAL RESPONSE

The patient's P waves measured 0.3 mV with the atrial sensitivity programmed to 0.3 mV. The atrial sensitivity was increased to 0.15 mV, which eliminated the atrial undersensing. No further inappropriate atrial pacing or safety pacing was observed.

13 | DDI Pacing Mode

DEVICE: Boston Scientific Essentio MRI L111 DC PM

PATIENT: A 59-year-old male received a dual-chamber pacemaker for intermittent AV block. The patient was hospitalized for a repeat procedure of an aortic root and arch replacement. The ECG tracing below (**Figure 13a**) was obtained at the bedside in the postoperative period. The bedside nurse requested a device interrogation due to inappropriate pacing. Programmed parameters are shown in **Figure 13b**. The EGM is shown in **Figure 13c**. What would explain the findings in the ECG tracing?

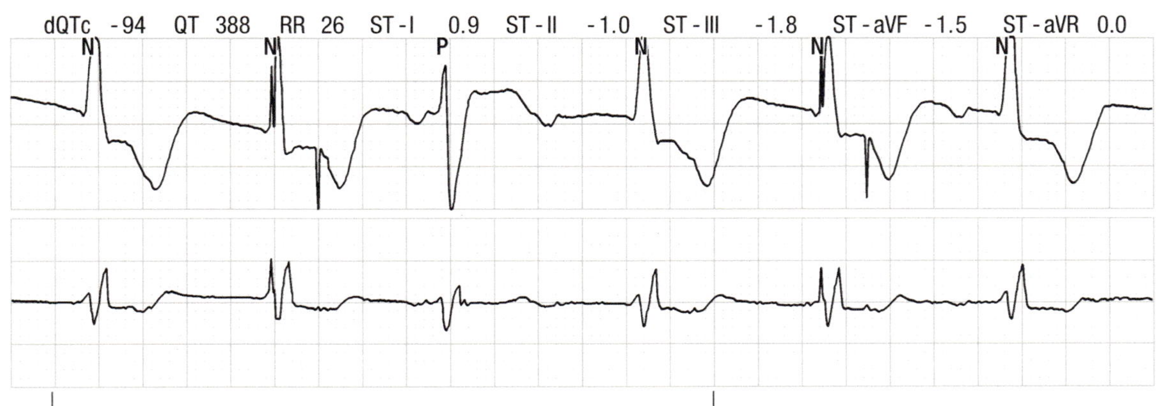

Figure 13a.

Brady			
Settings			
Mode	DDI	**Output**	
Lower Rate Limit	60 ppm	●A	Trend 3.5 V @ 0.4 ms
Paced AV Delay	210 ms	■V	Trend 3.5 V @ 0.4 ms
A-Refractory (PVARP)	280 ms	**Sensitivity**	
V-Refractory (VRP)	250 ms	●A	Fixed 0.25 mV
PVARP after PVC	400 ms	■V	Fixed 2.5 mV
AV Search +	Off	**Leads**	
Blanking		●A	
A-Blank after V-Pace	125 ms	Pace	Bipolar
A-Blank after V-Sense	45 ms	Sense	Bipolar
V-Blank after A-Pace	65 ms	Safety Switch	On
Magnet Response	Pace Async	■V	
Noise Response	DOO	Pace	Bipolar
Rate Enhancements		Sense	Bipolar
Rate Smoothing		Safety Switch	On
Down	Off %	**Rate Adaptive Pacing**	
Rate Hysteresis		Minute Ventilation	Passive
Hysteresis Offset	Off ppm	Accelerometer	Passive
		Minute Ventilation Sensor Settings	
		Minute Ventilation Sensor	Passive
		Excitation Current	320 µA
		Vector Selection	Auto Select
		Signal Artifact Monitor	On
		Minute Ventilation Sensor Status	
		Status	Initializing

Figure 13b.

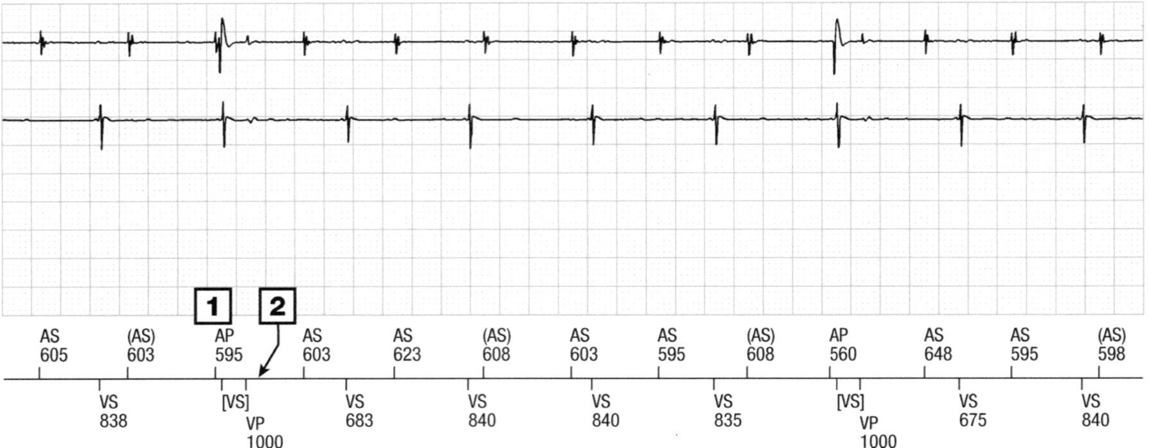

Figure 13c.

ANALYSIS

1. With the device programmed to the DDI mode, at [1] the AP and [VS] occur almost simultaneously, and the device labels the ventricular event as a VS. With the V-Blank after A-Pace programmed to 65 ms, the VS event occurs within the ventricular blanking period as evidenced by the 'VS' marker. A VP [2] is delivered at 210 ms.

2. Events falling within the postatrial ventricular blanking period (PAVBP) are ignored by the device, therefore, the VP [2] is still delivered at the programmed paced AV interval (210 ms).

CLINICAL RESPONSE

The device is functioning as programmed. The patient is in complete heart block with loss of AV synchrony. The nontracking mode of DDI was programmed to prevent tracking the fast atrial rate but is suboptimal given the inability to "track" and loss of AV synchrony.

14 | Functional Ventricular Undersensing

DEVICE: Boston Scientific Essentio MRI EL L131 DC PM

PATIENT: A 59-year-old male was hospitalized for a repeat procedure of an aortic root, arch, and valve replacement. Following surgery, an intermittent AV block was observed and a dual-chamber pacemaker was implanted. A suspicious ECG tracing was obtained via cardiac monitoring during the postoperative period (**Figure 14a**). The EGM recording corresponding to the event captured on telemetry is shown in **Figure 14b**.

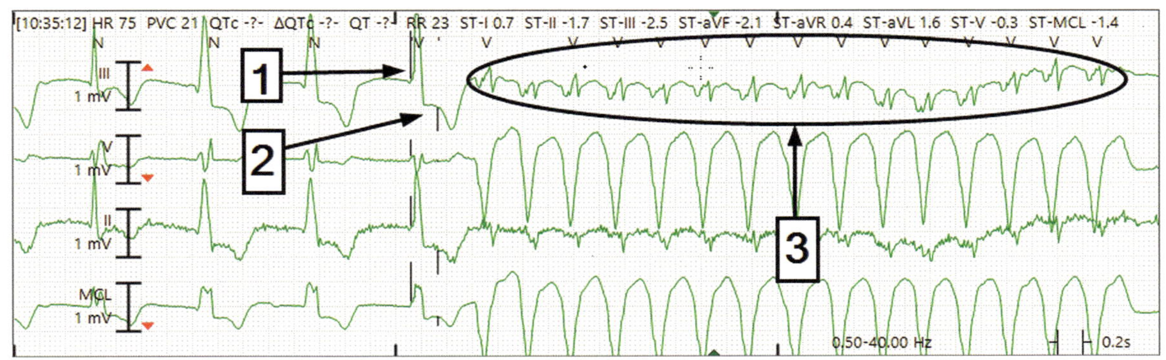

Figure 14a.

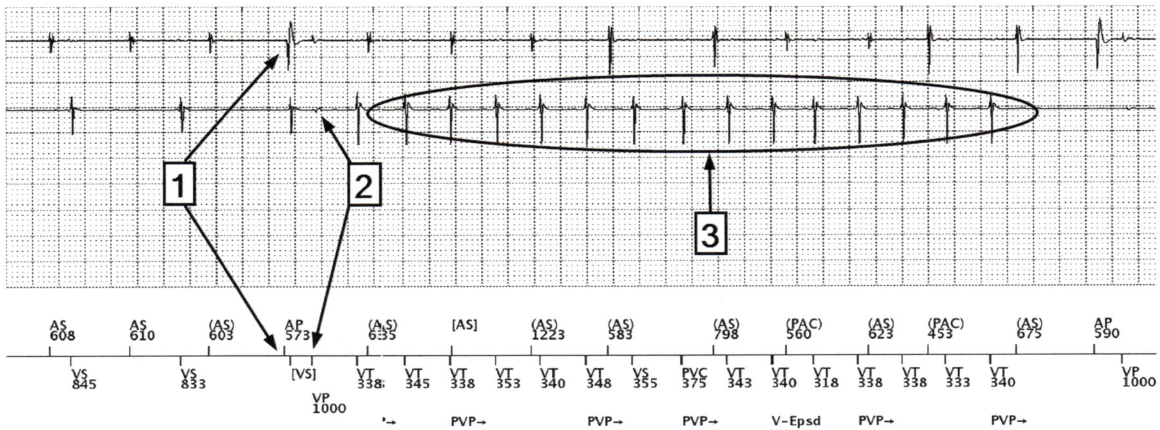

Figure 14b.

Brady	
Settings	
Mode	DDI
Lower Rate Limit	60 ppm
Paced AV Delay	210 ms
A-Refractory (PVARP)	280 ms
V-Refractory (VRP)	250 ms
PVARP after PVC	400 ms
AV Search +	Off
Blanking	
A-Blank after V-Pace	125 ms
A-Blank after V-Sense	45 ms
V-Blank after A-Pace	85 ms
Magnet Response	Pace Async
Noise Response	DOO

Figure 14c.

ANALYSIS

1. At the time of pacemaker implantation the patient was in sinus rhythm and the pacemaker mode was programmed DDI at 60 bpm. Pacemaker settings are shown in **Figure 14c**. Pacemaker timing interpretation is often difficult using ECG tracings alone. Using the corresponding EGM tracing, we are able to understand the event in detail. The beginning of the EGM shows evidence of heart block. DDI is a nontracking mode, but dual-chamber refractory and blanking periods are still enforced. The atrial timer ignores the refractory atrial sensed event (AS) and subsequently atrial paces AP. The atrial timer paces (1000 ms – 210 ms) 790 ms following the previous VS. At approximately the same time, an intrinsic ventricular beat [VS] falls into the V-Blank after A-Pace period [1].

2. The [VS] event is ignored by the ventricular timer and the device ventricular paces ventricular paces [2]. The ventricular timer paces 1000 ms following the previous VS. The VP event [2] is closely coupled to the [VS] event and appears to fall within what would be considered the vulnerable zone of ventricular repolarization.

3. The 15-beat run of ventricular ectopy [3] that ensues was most likely caused by ventricular pacing in vulnerable period.

CLINICAL RESPONSE

All lead testing was within normal limits. This sequence of events appears precipitated by the DDI programming mode in conjunction with AV dissociation. Fortunately, the recorded EGM was available for assessment. The programming mode was changed from DDI to DDD, which eliminated further occurrence of this phenomenon. The DDI mode is often chosen as a safe "backup" pacing mode among patients with atrial arrhythmias. This case illustrates how the DDI mode is not always benign.

15 | Atrial Sensed Events in Refractory Period

DEVICE: Medtronic Azure XT DR MRI W1DR01 DC PM

PATIENT: A 53-year-old patient with a history of recurrent syncope received his initial dual-chamber pacemaker at the age of 12. The patient's device was programmed DDI at 40 bpm to minimize ventricular pacing since the patient had a ventricular pace on the T wave in the setting of hypokalemia, which led to a ventricular arrhythmia. The patient has undergone multiple pulse generator changes for battery depletion. After the most recent generator change the following EGM was obtained. As demonstrated on this EGM, why are atrial events occurring in a refractory period?

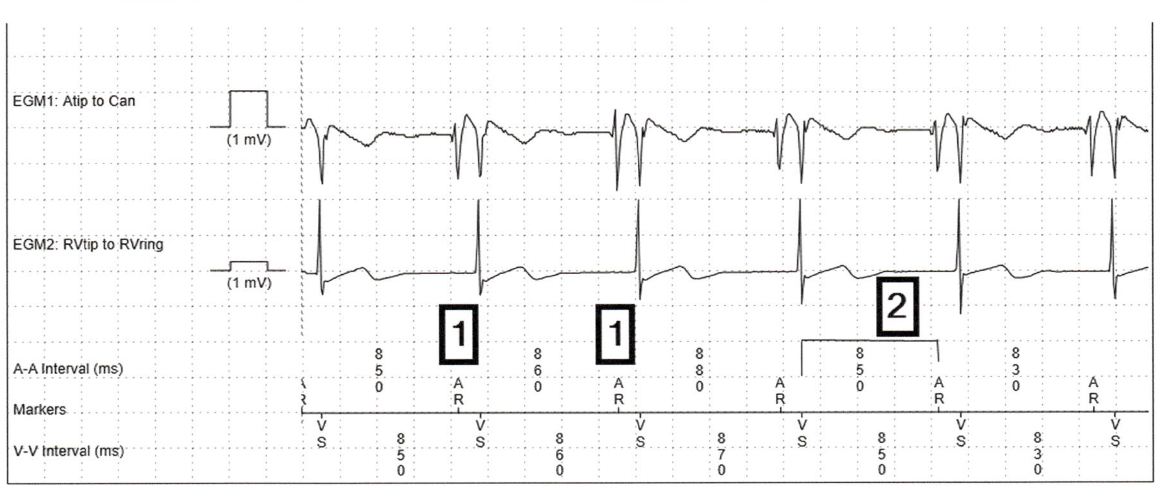

Figure 15a.

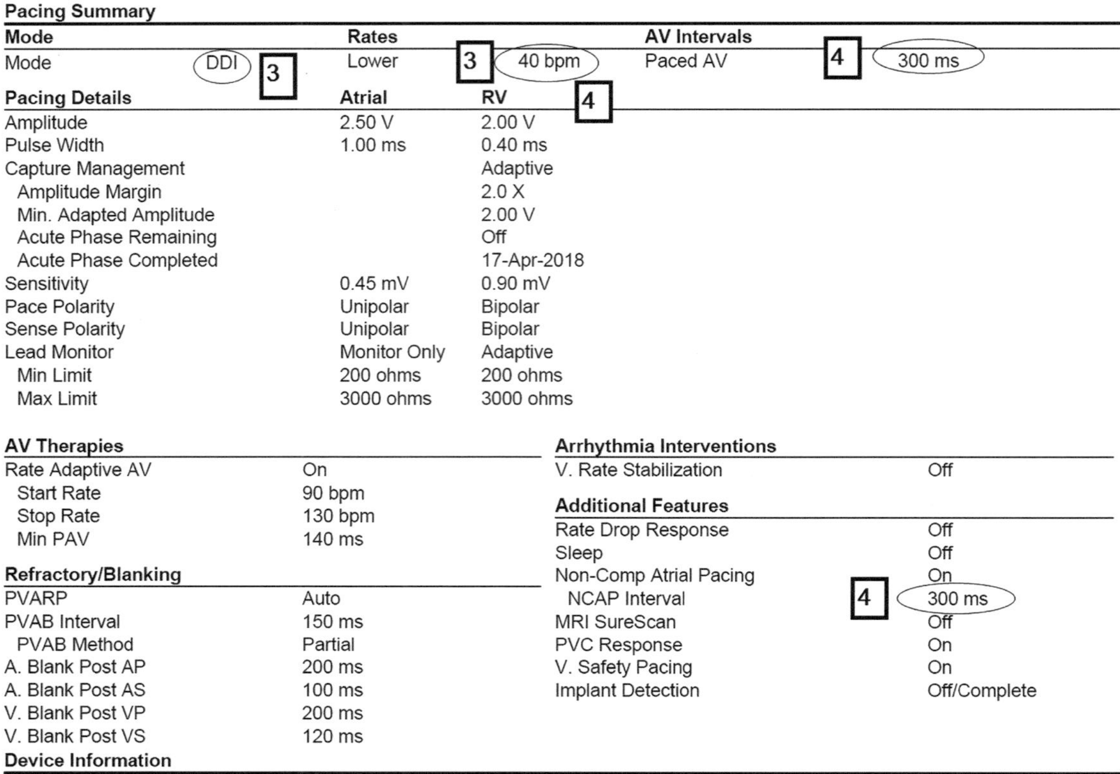

Pacing Summary

Mode		Rates		AV Intervals	
Mode	DDI **3**	Lower	**3** 40 bpm	Paced AV	**4** 300 ms

Pacing Details	Atrial	RV **4**
Amplitude	2.50 V	2.00 V
Pulse Width	1.00 ms	0.40 ms
Capture Management		Adaptive
Amplitude Margin		2.0 X
Min. Adapted Amplitude		2.00 V
Acute Phase Remaining		Off
Acute Phase Completed		17-Apr-2018
Sensitivity	0.45 mV	0.90 mV
Pace Polarity	Unipolar	Bipolar
Sense Polarity	Unipolar	Bipolar
Lead Monitor	Monitor Only	Adaptive
Min Limit	200 ohms	200 ohms
Max Limit	3000 ohms	3000 ohms

AV Therapies		Arrhythmia Interventions	
Rate Adaptive AV	On	V. Rate Stabilization	Off
Start Rate	90 bpm	**Additional Features**	
Stop Rate	130 bpm		
Min PAV	140 ms	Rate Drop Response	Off
		Sleep	Off
Refractory/Blanking		Non-Comp Atrial Pacing	On
PVARP	Auto	NCAP Interval	**4** 300 ms
PVAB Interval	150 ms	MRI SureScan	Off
PVAB Method	Partial	PVC Response	On
A. Blank Post AP	200 ms	V. Safety Pacing	On
A. Blank Post AS	100 ms	Implant Detection	Off/Complete
V. Blank Post VP	200 ms		
V. Blank Post VS	120 ms		
Device Information			

Figure 15b.

ANALYSIS

1. In **Figure 15a**, all the atrial events are falling into the postventricular atrial refractory period (PVARP) despite having a normal PR interval.

2. In Figure 15a, the V-to-A timing is roughly 740 ms, yet the intrinsic atrial events are consistently falling into the PVARP.

3. In **Figure 15b**, which shows the programmed parameters, note that the device is programmed to a DDI mode with a lower rate set to 40 bpm (1500-ms cycle length).

4. Since the patient is in the nontracking DDI mode, the maximum PVARP is calculated by taking the programmed lower rate limit of 1500 ms minus the programmed paced AV delay of 300 ms and the non-competitive atrial pacing interval (NCAP) of 300 ms, which gives you a PVARP of 900 ms. (NCAP is a feature that Medtronic utilizes within their devices to prevent pacing within the atrial refractory period, which could trigger an atrial tachycardia.)

CLINICAL RESPONSE

Despite this functionally long PVARP, the device is operating normally per the programmed parameters, which are exclusive to Medtronic devices. In a tracking mode with in the Medtronic: Adapta, Versa, Sensia, and Kappa devices, e.g., DDD, the device calculates the PVARP by taking the average R-to-R intervals and adding 30 bpm to give you a total calculated interval in ms. Then you take the total calculated interval and you subtract the sensed AV delay to get the maximum PVARP, which will never exceed 600 ms in a tracking mode, e.g., DDD. An example in a tracking mode would be the following: with an average R-to-R interval of 60 bpm, the addition of 30 bpm results in a rate of 90 bpm or a cycle length of 667 ms (60,000 ÷ 90 = 667 ms) minus a sensed AV delay of 150 ms, producing a total PVARP of 517 ms.

SUMMARY

Nontracking mode: PVARP = Lower rate – paced AV delay – NCAP

Tracking mode = PVARP = Total calculated interval – sensed AV delay

16 | Pseudo-Wenckebach Upper Rate Behavior

DEVICE: Medtronic Viva Quad XT DTBA1Q1 CRT-D

PATIENT: A 79-year-old patient with a history of heart failure with left ventricular systolic dysfunction, ventricular tachycardia and atrial arrhythmia currently has a CRT-D. The patient's underlying rhythm is third-degree atrioventricular block, and he is pacemaker-dependent. The patient's ejection fraction has increased from to 20% to 58% since CRT-D implant. The EGM in **Figure 16a** is observed during remote follow-up. Programmed parameters are shown in **Figure 16b**.

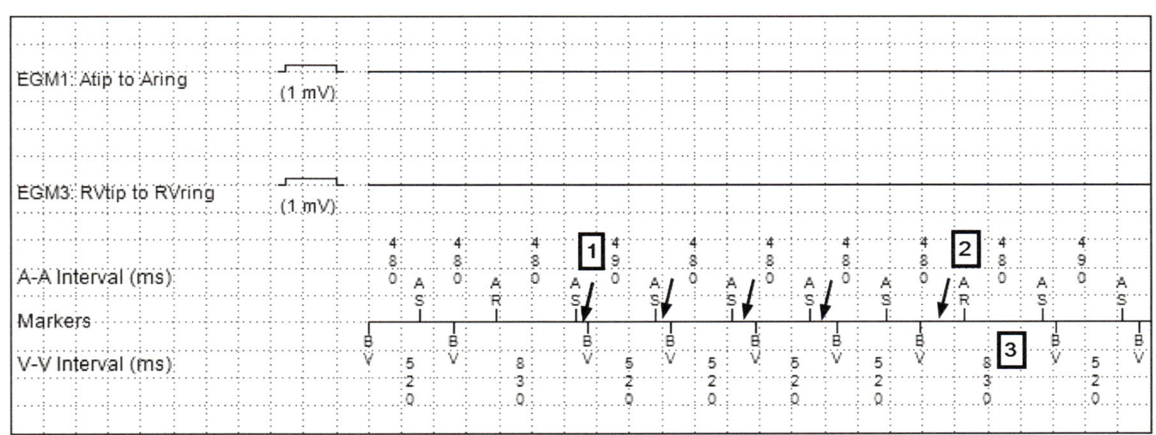

Figure 16a.

Pacing Summary

Mode		Rates		CRT	
Mode	DDDR	Lower	60 bpm	AdaptivCRT	Nonadaptive CRT
Mode Switch	171 bpm	Upper Track	115 bpm	V. Pacing	LV->RV
		Upper Sensor	115 bpm	V-V Pace Delay	0 ms
				Paced AV	130 ms
				Sensed AV	100 ms

Refractory/Blanking

PVARP	280 ms

Figure 16b.

1. The sensed AV interval is programmed at 100 ms and is observed in Figure 16a [1]. As the EGM progresses the AS to BV pace interval gradually increases above the programmed sensed AV interval (see black arrows). The BV pacing interval of 520 ms (115 bpm) is not changing due to the programmed upper tracking rate of 115 bpm. This combination results in slight shortening of BV-to-AS intervals. Most modern devices use a modified atrial based timing to not violate the programmed upper tracking rate.

2. Eventually the AS falls into the programmed postventricular atrial refractory period (PVARP), which is programmed to 280 ms and is labeled AR, seen at [2]. The AR event [2] does not trigger a BV paced event and the pattern continues.

3. This type of upper rate response is referred to as pacemaker Wenckebach or pseudo-Wenckebach.

CLINICAL RESPONSE

At the time of CRT implant, the patient's clinical condition warranted an upper tracking rate limited to 115 bpm. As the patient's condition improved following CRT implant, the patient's exercise tolerance improved. The patient's upper tracking rate was appropriately increased to 130 bpm.

17 | Pseudo-Wenckebach Upper Rate Behavior

DEVICE: Boston Scientific Cognis 100-D N119 CRT-D

PATIENT: A 78-year-old patient with an ischemic cardiomyopathy and impaired left ventricular systolic function who had undergone AV node ablation 7 years earlier to control symptoms related to paroxysmal atrial tachyarrhythmias and rapid ventricular response received a dual-chamber CRT-D device. Currently, he describes intermittent heart racing and fullness in his neck. The EGM below (**Figure 17a**) was obtained on a routine quarterly LATITUDE transmission. Rate histograms are shown in **Figure 17b**.

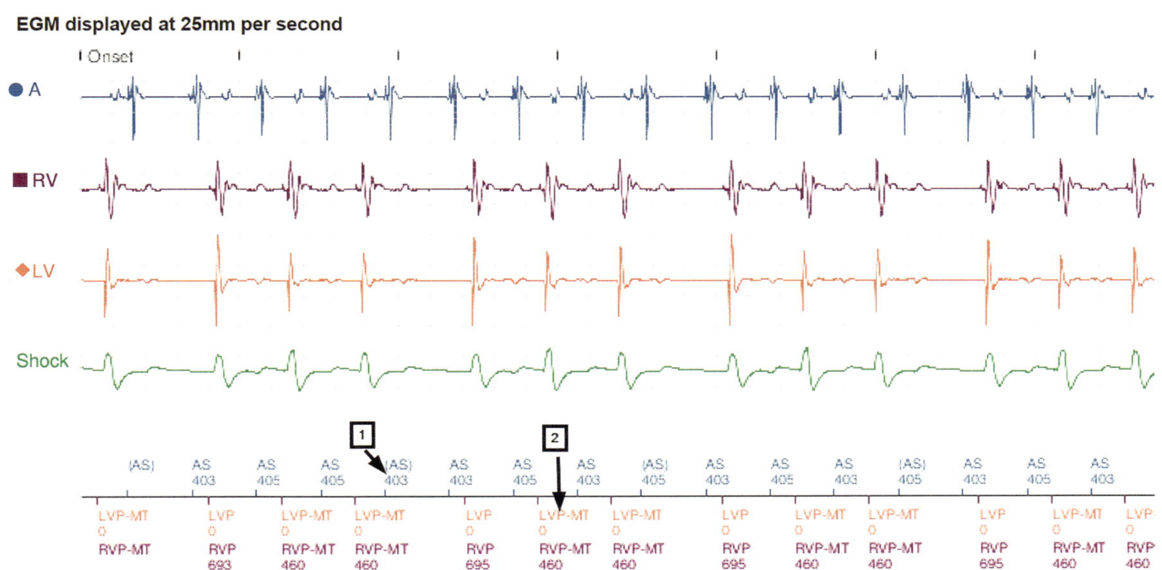

Figure 17a.

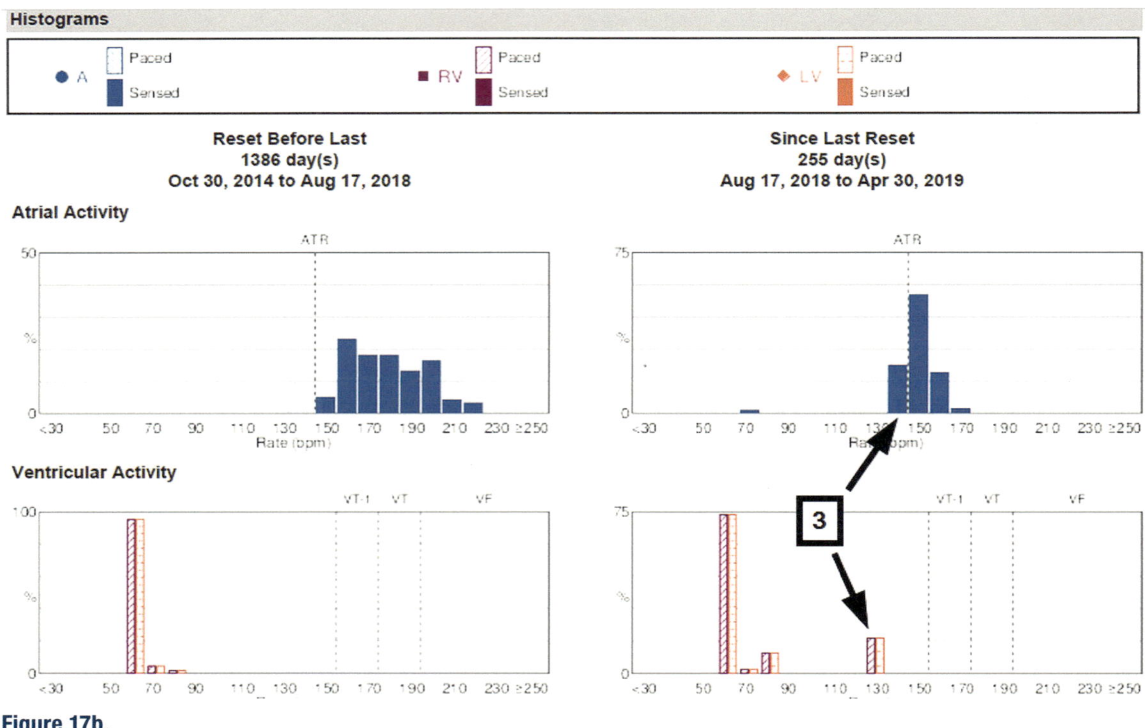

Figure 17b.

ANALYSIS

1. An atrial sensed beat falls into PVARP [1], resulting in this beat not being tracked and a subsequent dropped beat. The dropped beats occur in a recurrent pattern or "patterned beating" which is a hallmark of recognizing pseudo-Wenckebach upper rate behavior.

2. Bi-V pacing at maximum tracking rate (MTR) of 130 bpm ([2] LVP-MT). Sensed A-V delay is programmed fixed at 100 ms. Note the longer A-V delay, other than what is programmed for this tracked atrial event, so that the MTR is not violated.

3. Comparing the two atrial histograms, the atrial rate on average has slowed over time, with nearly 20% of the time falling below the mode switch rate of 150 bpm on the most recent histogram [3]. Due to this, the device has paced nearly 20% of the time at or near the MTR of 130 bpm, causing the symptoms the patient was experiencing. The symptoms were not from ventricular high rates (ventricular tachycardia), but rather as a result of tracking the atrial tachyarrhythmias as evidenced by the distribution of rates on the ventricular rate histogram.

CLINICAL RESPONSE

Due to the patient's longstanding atrial tachyarrhythmias, the device was programmed to VVIR, eliminating any chance of pacing inappropriately at MTR given the lack of atrial sensing and tracking in this pacing mode.

18 | Pseudo-Wenckebach Upper Rate Behavior

DEVICE: St. Jude Medical* Allure Quadra 3242 CRT-P

PATIENT: An active 46-year-old patient with a history of significant left ventricular dysfunction and AV block following ablation for AV node reentry tachycardia underwent CRT-P implant. The patient called the device clinic and reported symptoms of fatigue with activity and sent a remote transmission. The EGM tracing from the remote follow-up is shown below in **Figure 18a**. A list of pertinent programmed parameters is shown in **Figure 18b**. What programming changes would be appropriate?

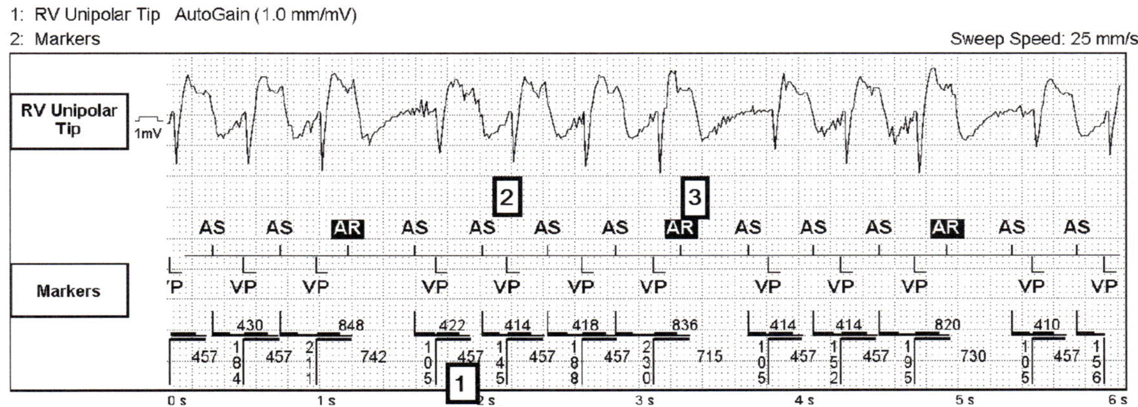

Figure 18a.

Mode	DDD
Lower rate	60
Maximum tracking rate	130 bpm
Maximum sensor rate	130 bpm
Paced AV	100 ms
Sensed AV	100 ms
Mode	250 ms

Figure 18b.

---

*St. Jude Medical is now Abbott.

1. Ventricular pacing has a distinct pattern of regular timing at 130 bpm [1] with periodic interruptions. The MTR is programmed at 130 bpm.

2. The intrinsic atrial rhythm is fairly regular at approximately 142 bpm [2], therefore ventricular pacing incrementally lags the atrial sensed events by extending the AS to VP interval. This occurs when the device continues to track the intrinsic atrial rhythm without violating the MTR of 130 bpm (457 ms).

3. The VP to AS decreases as a result of the increasing AS to VP interval. When the VP to AS interval falls within the programmed postventricular atrial refractory period (PVARP), the atrial event is marked as being refractory (AR). Atrial events falling into PVARP will not be tracked by the device [3]. Ventricular tracking then resumes when the next atrial event falls into the atrial alert period. This type of upper rate behavior is referred to as pacemaker Wenckebach or pseudo-Wenckebach. The "patterned beating" is characteristic of pseudo-Wenckebach behavior.

CLINICAL RESPONSE

Based on atrial rate histogram diagnostics, this patient's heart rate increased to a maximum of 155 bpm with exercise. The MTR was changed to 160 bpm. With a MTR of 160 bpm, the total atrial refractory period (TARP) should also be considered for programming adjustments. If the TARP (AVD + PVARP) is too long, the device will not be able to achieve the new MTR, and will create another upper rate behavior situation. In order to accommodate the MTR of 160 bpm, rate responsive AV delays and rate responsive PVARP were also programmed on in order to minimize the length of the TARP interval as the patient's heart rate increases.

19 | His Pacing Threshold at Implant

DEVICE: Medtronic Azure XT DR MRI W1DR01 DC PM

PATIENT: A 78-year-old female patient undergoes dual-chamber pacemaker implant for symptomatic second-degree AV block (Wenckebach), blocked PACs and intermittent junctional rhythm seen on a Holter monitor. This patient also had an underlying prolonged A-V delay of 380 ms. The right ventricular lead was placed in the His bundle position due to anticipated frequent right ventricular pacing in an effort to mimic normal ventricular activation, minimizing chance of developing pacing induced cardiomyopathy. The patient's 12-lead ECG is shown in **Figure 19a** and a tracing obtained during device evaluation is shown in **Figure 19b**.

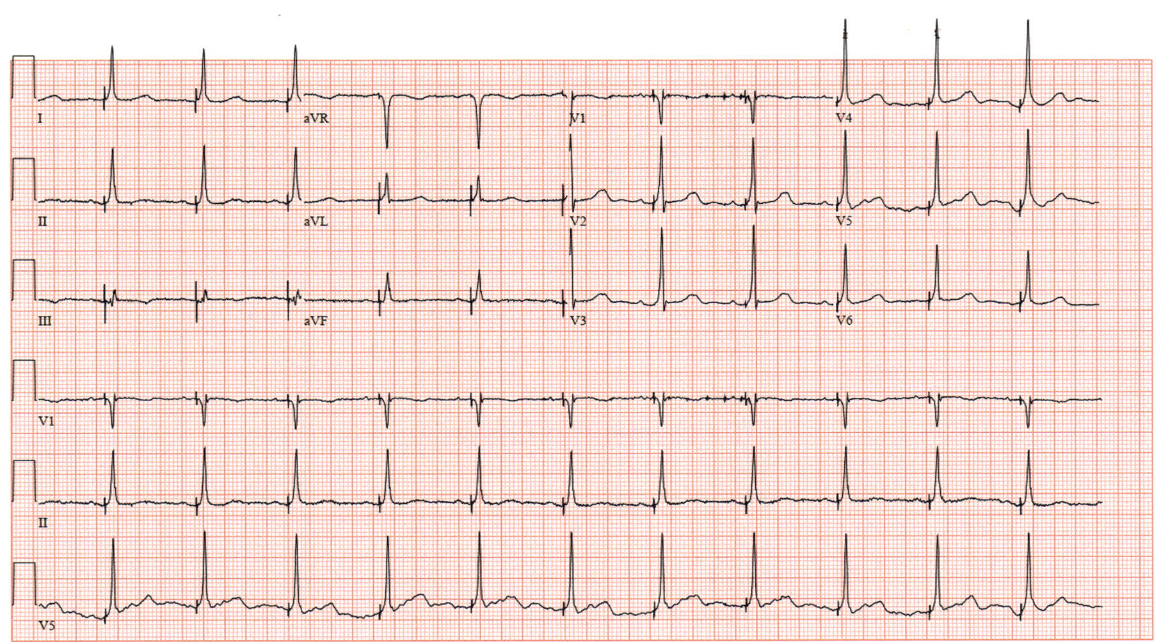

Figure 19a.

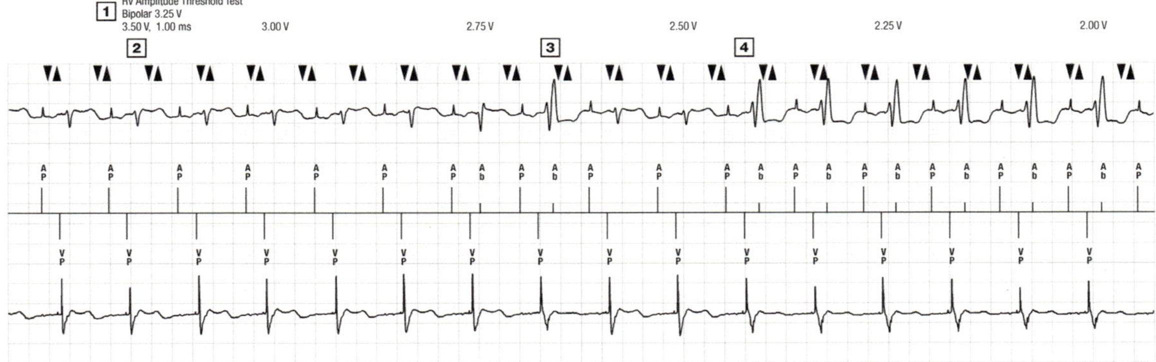

Figure 19b.

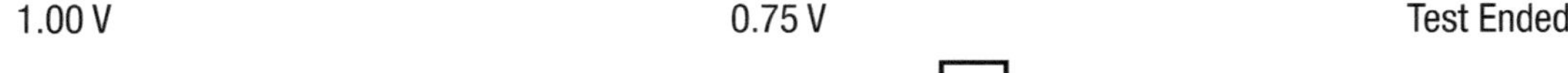

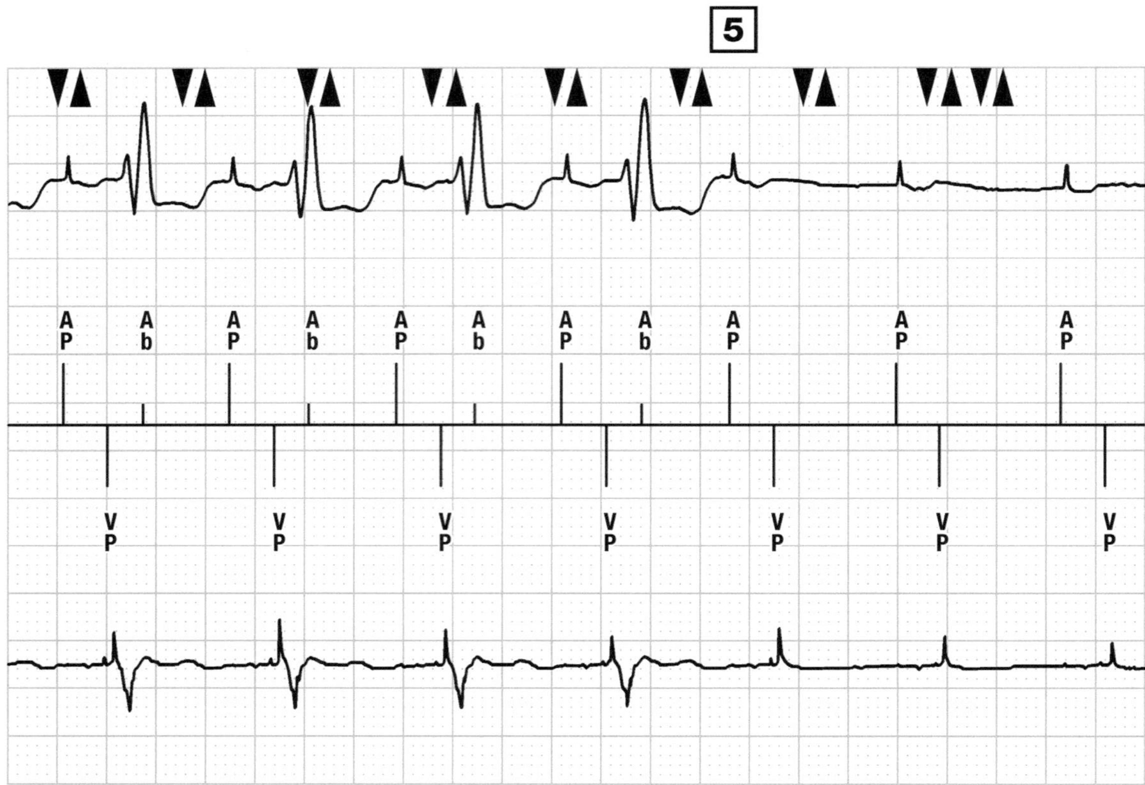

Figure 19c.

ANALYSIS

1. The tracing in Figure 19b represents an RV threshold test of a Medtronic 3830 SelectSecure MRI SureScan lead implanted in the His bundle position.

2. With His bundle pacing, the objective is to obtain a narrow (<120 ms) QRS complex or one that is identical to patients intrinsic QRS. A narrow, normal paced QRS with His pacing with isoelectric interval between the pacing stimulus and the QRS is considered selective pacing. In selective His bundle pacing, the pacing impulse is capturing the His bundle only and the impulse then conducts to the right and left bundle branches, initiating ventricular contraction. As the proximal conduction system is insulated, an isoelectric interval is seen with selective His bundle pacing. A narrow QRS complex from a pacing impulse in the His position without an isoelectric interval is considered non-selective His pacing. It is considered non-selective because the pacing impulse is capturing the His bundle as well as the local myocardium around the His bundle. As the output is reduced, only local myocardial capture occurs with QRS widening.

3. Threshold test can be recognized by the decrementing voltage by 0.25 V every three impulses until manually ending the test. The test was performed at a pulse width of 1 ms.

4. Starting at 3.5 V/1 ms [1], note that the RV paced QRS is narrow, approximately 120 ms [2]. As threshold test continues and the voltage decreased, there is one pacing impulse at 2.75 V/1 ms, which resulted in a widened QRS [3]; therefore, the non-selective His pacing threshold is 3 V/1 ms. At 2.5 V/1 ms, the QRS becomes consistently widened to approximately 200 ms [4].

5. Complete loss of ventricular capture is at 0.75 V/1 ms with patient becoming intermittently dependent during this implant procedure [5] (**Figure 19c**). Therefore, ventricular threshold is 1 V/1 ms.

CLINICAL RESPONSE

With His bundle pacing, unique programming parameters need to be considered. These may include RV amplitude, pulse width, and other automatic device functions that may change these parameters. In this case, as noted in the tracing above, non-selective His bundle capture or ventricular myocardium-only capture can be achieved by either increasing or decrease the pacing impulse voltage. Without awareness of His bundle pacing and its intended clinical response, a clinician may run a RV threshold test and note a RV threshold of 1 V/1 ms and program the RV amplitude to 2 V/1 ms accounting for a safety margin that is twice the threshold. If one were to do this, an RV amplitude of 2 V/1 ms would result in myocardium-only RV pacing and defeat the purpose of His bundle pacing. Automatic thresholds should be turned off when conduction system pacing is intended.

20 | Crosstalk Oversensing on Ventricular Channel with His Pace/Sense Lead in RV Port

DEVICE: Medtronic Advisa DR MRI A2DR01 DC PM

PATIENT: A 47-year-old patient received a heart transplant after viral myocarditis progressed to heart failure with an ejection fraction of 16% and LVAD placement. After transplant, the patient was in complete heart block with a sinus rate of 85 bpm and junctional escape rhythm at 65 bpm as shown in **Figure 20a**. The patient was implanted with a dual-chamber pacemaker. Within the transplanted heart, the ventricular lead is a bipolar lead with His bundle placement. The atrial lead is bipolar and placed in the atrium of the transplanted heart. Consider the presenting EGM from the hospital follow-up the day after implant shown in **Figure 20b**.

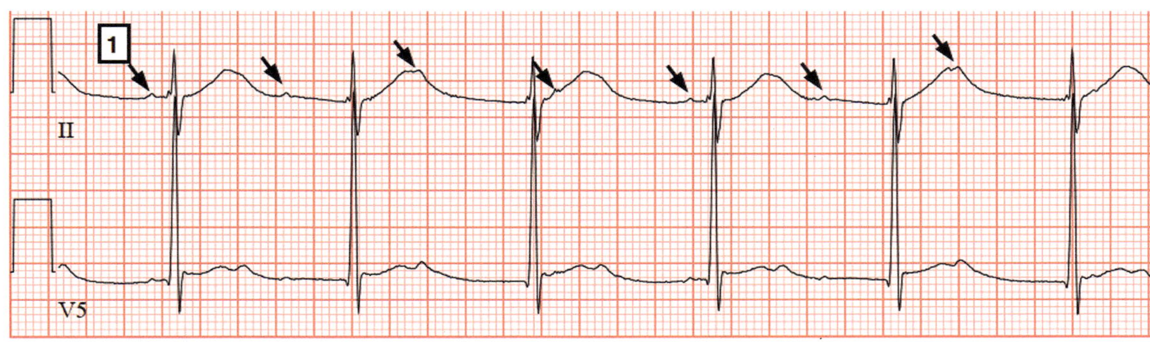

Figure 20a.

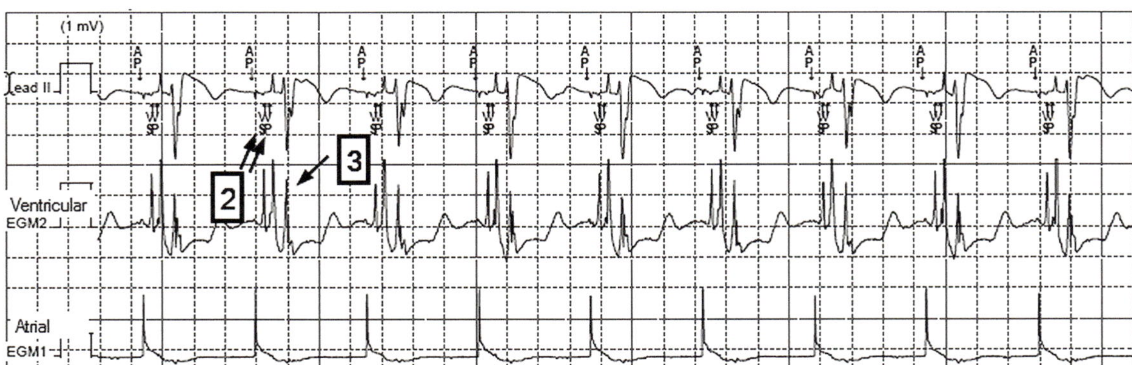

Figure 20b.

ANALYSIS

1. ECG strip taken after heart transplant before pacemaker placement is shown in Figure 20a. Sinus P waves are detectable [1] at ~85 bpm while the ventricular escape rhythm is ~65 bpm.

2. The day after pacemaker implantation, the presenting EGM is shown Figure 20b. The device is programmed AAIR ⟷ DDDR 70 to 130 bpm. The EGM shows atrial pacing at 85 bpm with ventricular oversensing of the atrial complex. Leads placed for His bundle pacing have greater potential for oversensing P waves due to His lead proximity to the atrium. The VS event following the AS falls into the atrial cross talk alert period and is followed by the ventricular safety pace, VP.

3. The actual ventricular QRS complex [3] is not sensed because it falls into the ventricular blanking postventricular pace period.

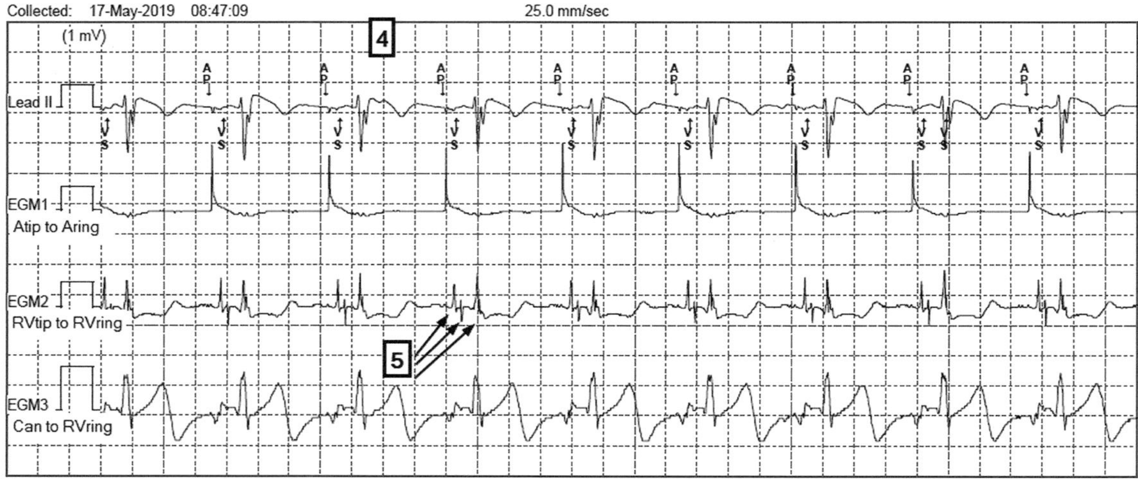

Figure 20c.

4. When the patient is atrial paced (AAI) the patient demonstrates intact AV conduction [4] as shown in **Figure 20c**. Following heart transplant, the patient demonstrated what appeared to be complete AV block as shown in Figure 20a. However, the native P waves [1] are actually from the base of the native heart with a junctional escape from the transplanted heart. Pacing via the newly implanted atrial pacing lead placed in the transplanted donor atrium intrinsically conducts.

5. The EGM2 is the bipolar RV lead with His placement. This EGM clearly shows electrical activity associated with the atrial, His, and ventricular depolarization.

CLINICAL RESPONSE

The intact AV conduction of the transplanted heart allowed the patient to be programmed in AAI mode. This eliminated the crosstalk and avoided His lead oversensing of the atrium.

21 | Pseudo Undersensing in Leadless Pacemaker

DEVICE: Medtronic Micra VR TCP MC1VR01 SC PM

PATIENT: A 90-year-old female with episodic pauses and syncope underwent leadless pacemaker implantation. During the implantation procedure, the following electrogram was obtained. An R-wave measurement could not be reliably obtained.

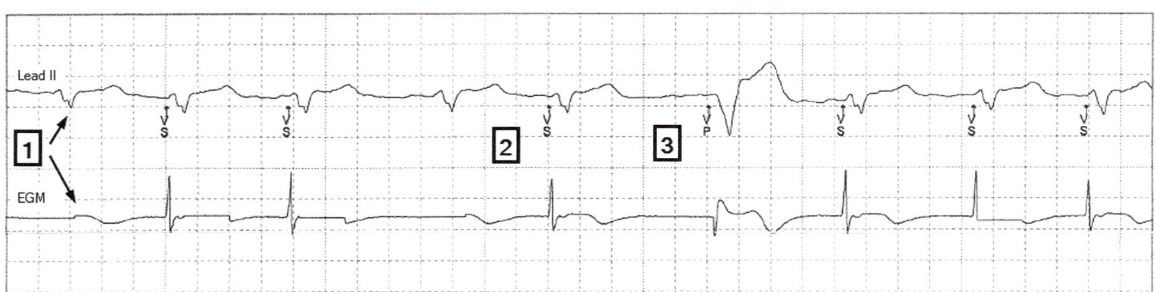

Figure 21.

ANALYSIS

1. The tracing shows electrograms from a leadless pacemaker device. The top tracing is a surface recording with superimposed event markers. The tracing in **Figure 21** is the intracardiac recordings from the device. We notice that for some beats there are missing intracardiac deflections [1] even though corresponding surface ECG tracing shows a QRS complex.

2. Some beats have a reasonable R wave below the corresponding QRS complex [2]. The R wave must be above the set sensitivity as the device recognizes the event and a sensed event (VS) is declared on the marker channel. When the ventricular rate falls below the programmed rate of 60 bpm, the device delivers a pacing pulse [3], resulting in electrical capture of the myocardium.

3. The Medtronic leadless pacemaker communicates with the programmer using radiofrequency telemetry. The header is often placed over the heart, and the number of green bars is noted to understand the signal strength. Intermittent loss of telemetry signal will result in loss of intracardiac electrograms without affecting the surface ECG. This is normal function of the device and pacemaker should not be repositioned for under-sensed R waves.

CLINICAL RESPONSE

The findings were reviewed with the electrophysiologist and were confirmed as pseudo-undersensing due to intermittent loss of telemetry. Following the change in the header position, the R waves were consistently above 10 mV, and the threshold was 0.25 mV/0.24 ms. The device was deployed at the current location, and the procedure was completed with any adverse events.

22 | Remote Alert Follow-Up

DEVICE: Boston Scientific Essentio L101 DC PM

PATIENT: A 69-year-old patient with atrial fibrillation underwent aortic valve replacement. Following surgery, conduction system disease and pauses with intermittent AV were observed. The patient underwent implantation of a dual-chamber pacemaker. Consider the following alert from remote follow-up in **Figure 22a**.

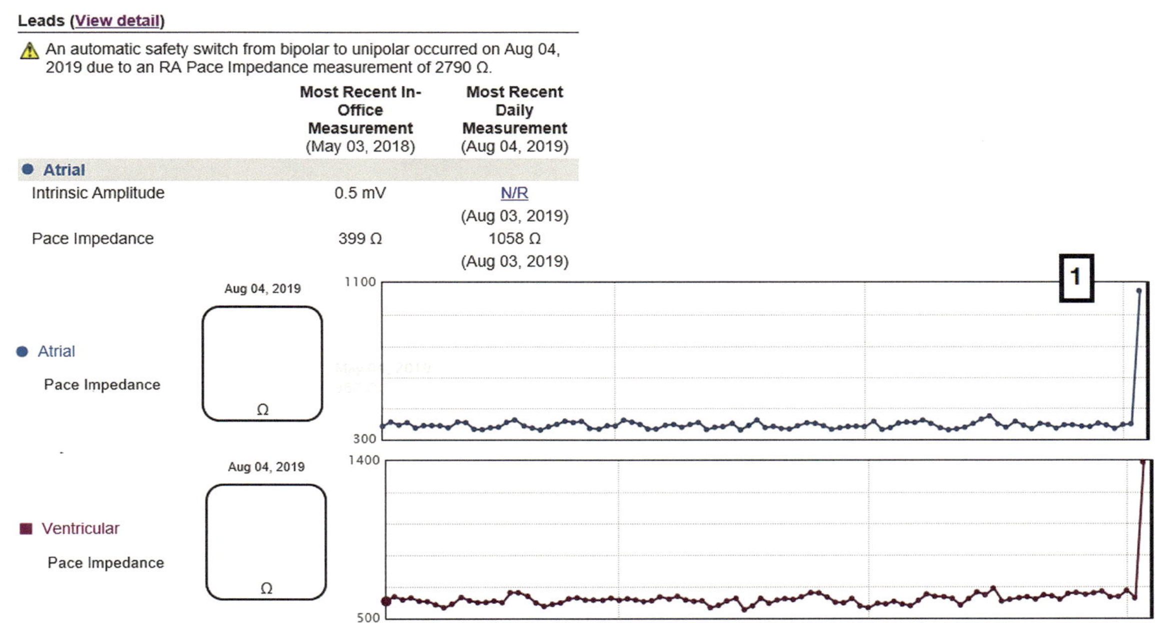

Figure 22a.

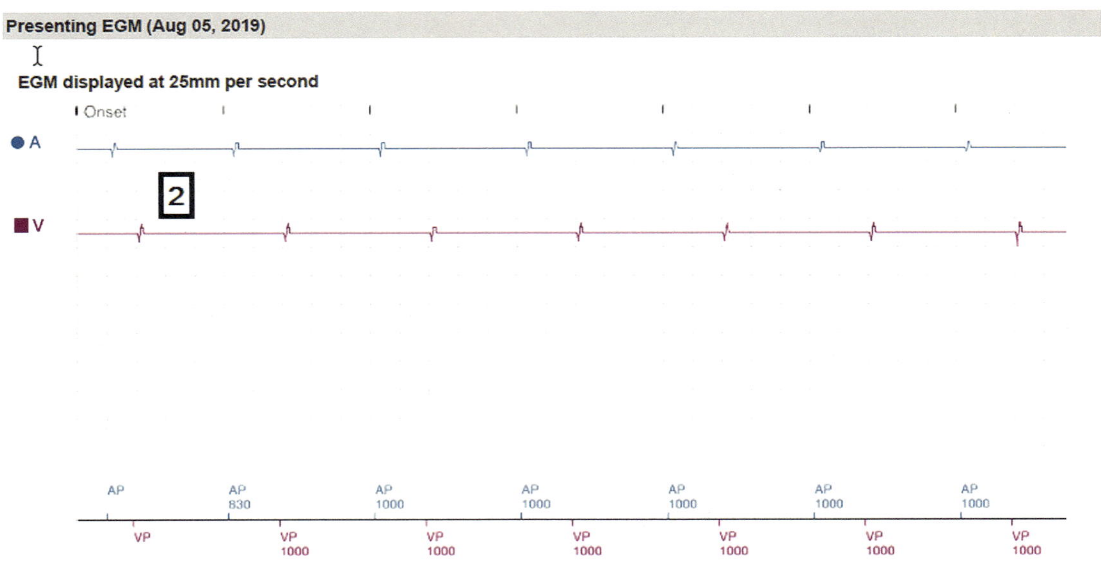

Figure 22b.

ANALYSIS

1. The remote alerts us to a high atrial impedance measurement with the safety switch of polarity from bipolar to unipolar. The atrial lead impedance trend clearly shows an abrupt change in the atrial impedance [1]. This is concerning but not an unusual finding. There was no alert for the ventricular impedance, but we observe a similar rise in the ventricular impedance trend.

2. The presenting EGM in **Figure 22b** is unremarkable, showing dual-chamber pacing at a lower rate of 60 bpm [2]. The patient was previously known to be in atrial fibrillation.

3. This remote follow-up also reports two new ventricular tachycardia events as shown in **Figure 22c**. The first ventricular event, V-12, shown in Figure 22c begins with a more organized tachycardia rhythm [3]. Both the events show ventricular fibrillation initiated by ventricular ectopic beats. The second ventricular event, V-13, is less organized with intermittent undersensing, and atrial and ventricular pacing [4]. The lead impedance changes on both the leads and lack of a sensed electrical activity on the atrial lead point to something ominous.

V-12: Aug 03, 2019 21:15, VT (V>A), A Rate: 48 bpm, V Rate: 235 bpm

EGM displayed at 25mm per second

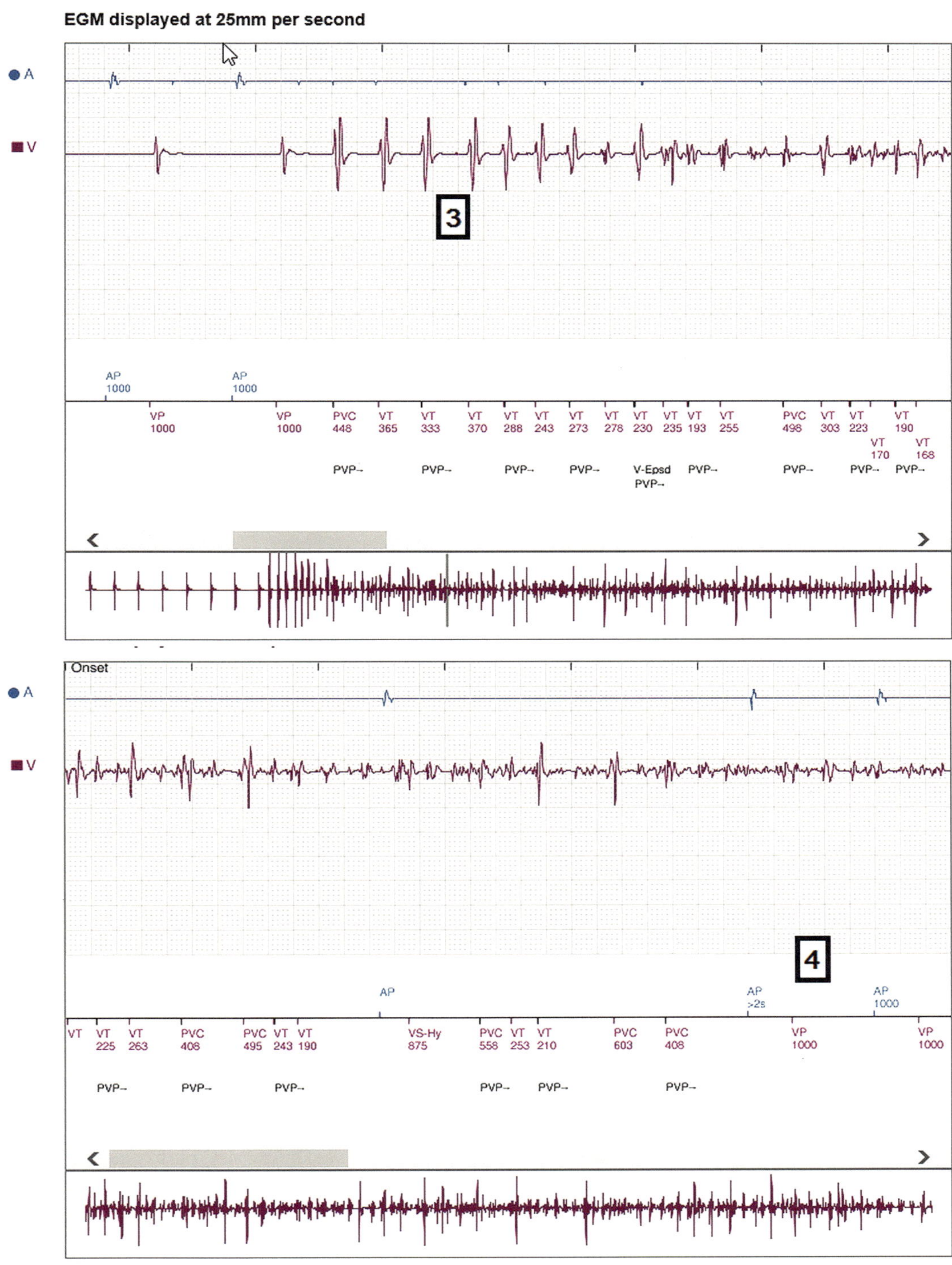

Figure 22c.

The lead alert and ventricular episodes reported in this remote report necessitate follow-up with an assessment of the patient. The device nurse was unable to reach the patient or the alternate patient contact by phone. The patient's primary care physician was consulted, and it was decided to contact the local emergency responders. Unfortunately, the patient was found by the police deceased in his home. Increase in lead impedance trends, lack of sensed electrical activity, and recording of ventricular arrhythmias before the last remote transmission all point to patient's demise.

23 | Promoting Intrinsic Ventricular Conduction

DEVICE: St. Jude Medical* Ellipse DR 2411-36Q DC ICD

PATIENT: A 65-year-old patient underwent dual-chamber ICD implantation for ischemic cardiomyopathy and symptomatic bradycardia. In the EGM shown in **Figure 23a**, how would you interpret the VIP function and its success in promoting intrinsic AV conduction with given programmed parameters (**Figure 23b**)?

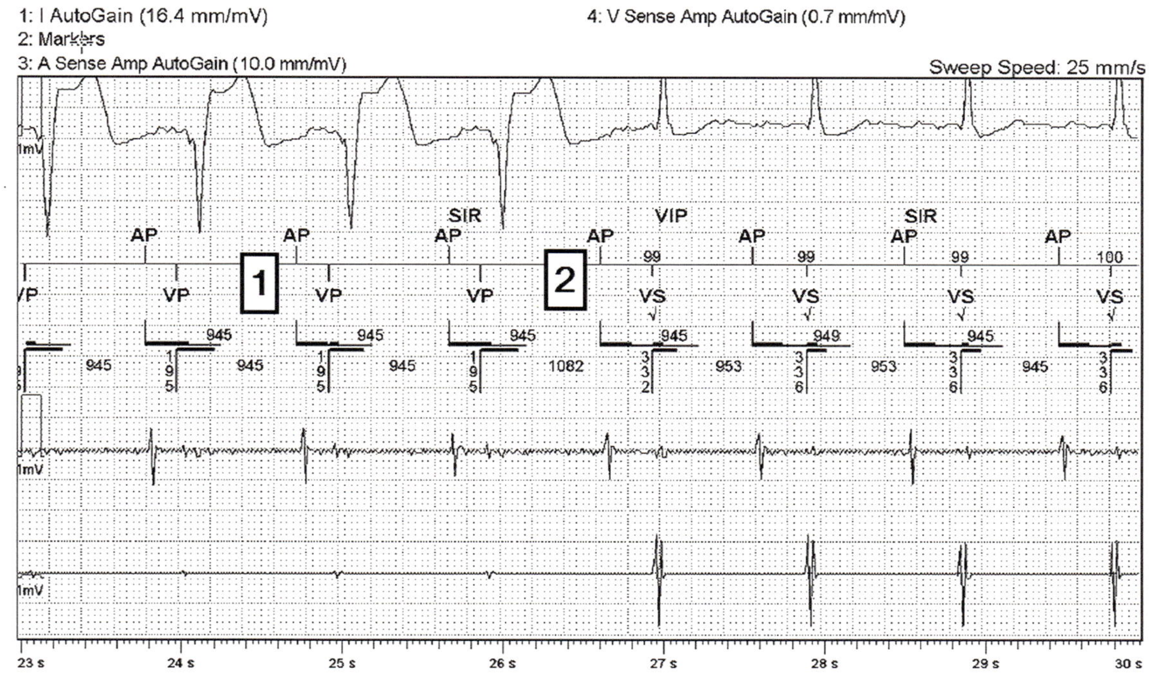

Figure 23a.

Basic Operation		Refractories & Blanking	
Mode	DDDR	PVARP	275 ms
Magnet Response	Normal	Post-Vent. Atrial Blanking	60 ms
V. Noise Reversion Mode	Pacing Off	Rate Responsive PVARP/V Ref	High
Episodal Pacing Mode	DDI	Shortest PVARP/V Ref	225 ms
Sensor	On	A/V Pace Refractory	190/220 ms
Threshold (Measured Avg.)	Auto (+0.0) (2.0)	A/V Sense Refractory	93/125 ms
Slope	8	Ventricular Blanking	52 ms
Max Sensor Rate	130 bpm	Ventricular Safety Standby	On
Reaction Time	Fast	Arrhythmia Unhiding	3 intervals
Recovery Time	Medium	PVC Response	Atrial Pace
		PMT Response	Atrial Pace
Rates		PMT Detection Rate	110 bpm
Base Rate	60 bpm		
Rest Rate	Off	**AT/AF Detection & Response**	
Max Sensor Rate	130 bpm	Auto Mode Switch	DDIR
Max Track Rate	130 bpm	A. Tachycardia Detection Rate	170 bpm
Hysteresis Rate	Off	AMS Base Rate	60 bpm
2:1 Block Rate	160 bpm	AF Suppression™	Off

Delays

Paced AV Delay		200 ms
Sensed AV Delay	3	150 ms
Rate Responsive AV Delay		Off
Ventricular Intrinsic Preference (VIP®)		On
VIP® Extension		180 ms
Search Interval		1 min
Search Cycles		1
Negative AV Hysteresis/Search		Off

Figure 23b.

ANALYSIS

1. The first three beats show AP VP at 65 bpm with the programmed A-V delay of 200 bpm.

2. After the fourth paced QRS complex, VIP extended the A-V delay by an additional 180 ms, allowing for intrinsic ventricular conduction with an A-R interval of 336 ms.

3. VIP can be programmed to extend A-V delay up to an additional 200 ms (max AV delay of 450 ms), with a search interval up to every 30 minutes or as frequent as every 30 seconds. It can also be programmed to search for 1 to 3 consecutive cycles. These features provide flexible programmability to promote intrinsic A-V conduction.

CLINICAL RESPONSE

Promoting intrinsic A-V conduction can benefit a patient by limiting RV pacing that may induce left ventricular systolic dysfunction and with clinical signs of heart failure. During follow-up encounters, RV pacing percentage will have to be monitored to assess the effectiveness of the VIP algorithm.

24 | Atrial Preference Pacing

DEVICE: Medtronic Evera XT DR DDBB1D1 DC ICD

PATIENT: A 73-year-old patient with ischemic cardiomyopathy is implanted with a dual-chamber ICD for paroxysmal ventricular tachycardia. The presenting EGM (**Figure 24a**) is from routine remote follow-up. What feature of this EGM is unique?

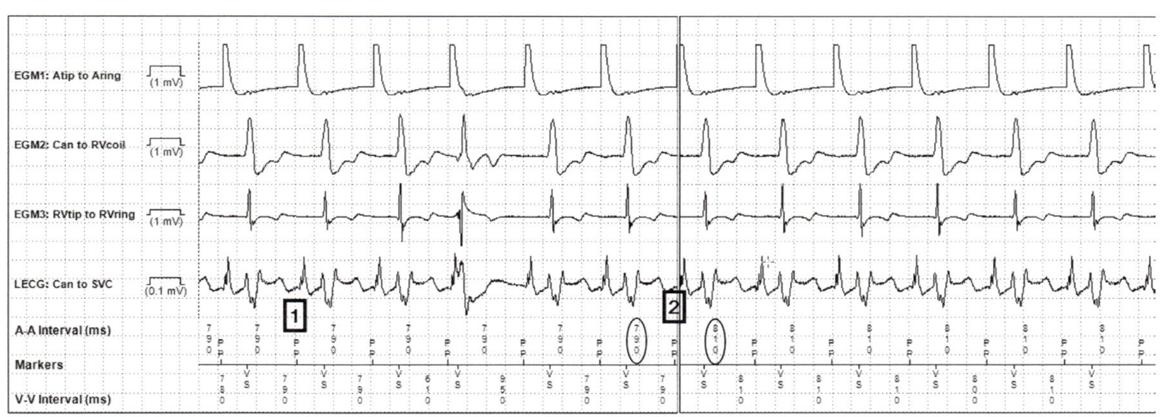

Figure 24a.

ANALYSIS

1. The atrial marker channel PP [1] is Medtronic's annotation for proactive pace (PP). This indicates the Atrial Preference Pacing™ (APP) feature is programmed on, as shown in **Figure 24b**. The APP feature is designed to maximize atrial pacing percentage in order to reduce the incidence of atrial tachyarrhythmias. With APP, when an atrial sensed event occurs, the device decrements the atrial paced interval by the programmed interval decrement (50 ms). The decrement in atrial pacing interval is repeated until reaching a paced rhythm that is faster than the intrinsic rate.

Mode		Rates		AV Intervals	
Mode	AAIR<=>DDDR	Lower	60 bpm	Paced AV	180 ms
Mode Switch	171 bpm	Upper Track	130 bpm	Sensed AV	150 ms
		Upper Sensor	130 bpm		

Arrhythmia Interventions	
A. Rate Stabilization	On
Maximum Rate	100 bpm
Interval Percentage Increment	25 %
A. Preference Pacing	On
Maximum Rate	100 bpm
Interval Decrement	50 ms
Search Beats	10

Figure 24b.

2. The increased rate is sustained for a programmable number of beats (Search Beats) after which the atrial interval is increased 20 ms in search of the next intrinsic beat [2]. In this case, the interval was increased by 810 ms; 810 ms – 790 ms = 20 ms. If no intrinsic beat is found, it continues to slow the rate by 20 ms intervals until an intrinsic beat occurs. This algorithm results in a controlled increase or decrease in atrial pacing intervals slightly above the intrinsic rate.

CLINICAL RESPONSE

The effectiveness of the algorithm is demonstrated by the diagnostic atrial histograms. The patient is atrial paced over 96% of the time (**Figure 24c**). The normal distribution of atrial pacing rates suggests dynamic and controlled pacing slightly above the intrinsic rate.

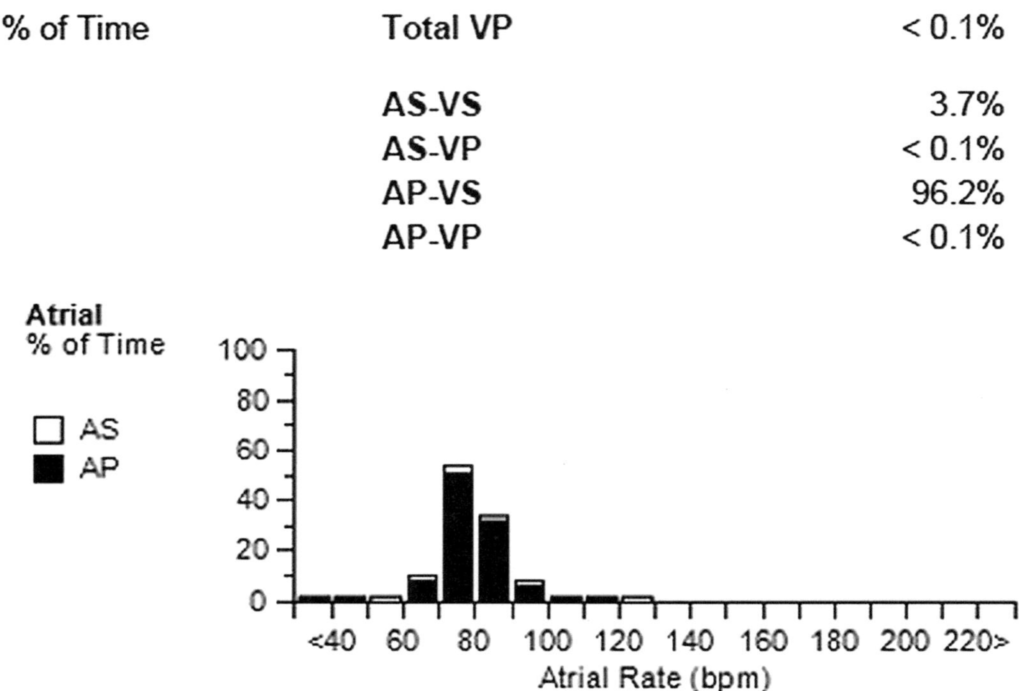

Figure 24c.

25 | Rate Drop Response

DEVICE: Medtronic Advisa DR MRI A2DR01 DC PM

PATIENT: A 32-year-old patient reported multiple episodes of syncope and presyncope. The patient underwent tilt-table testing, which revealed neurocardiogenic syncope with a strong cardioinhibitory component. A cardiac loop recorder was implanted and it recorded an episode with a 35-second pause coincident with patient symptoms of syncope. The patient was subsequently implanted with a dual-chamber pacemaker with a Rate Drop Response feature. The following episode reported by routine remote monitoring illustrates a clinical example of how the Rate Drop feature functions.

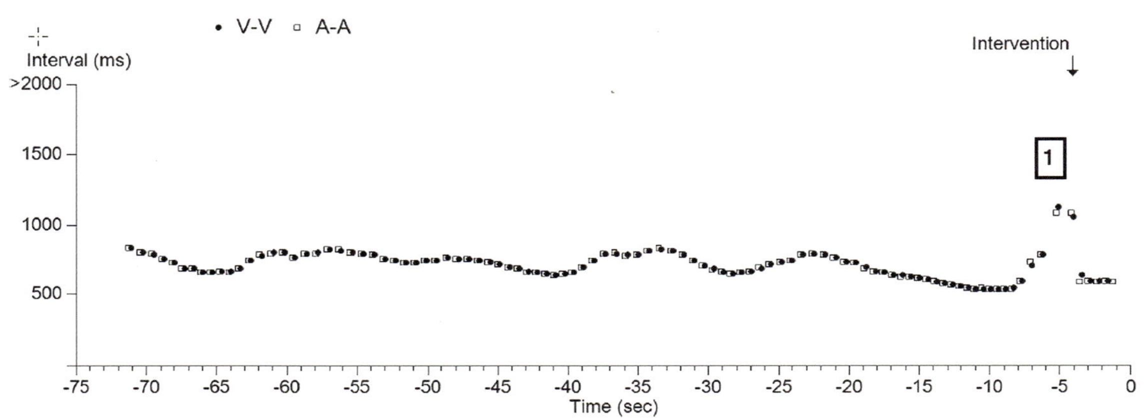

Figure 25a.

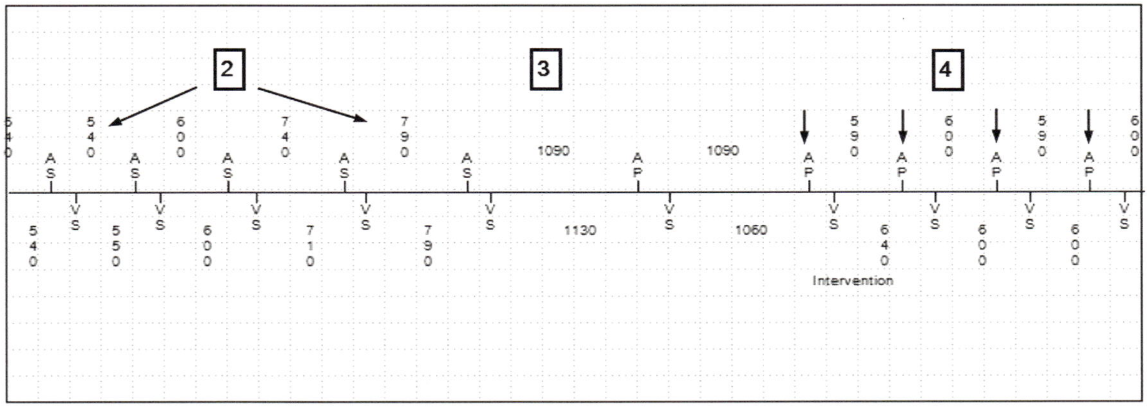

Figure 25b.

1. It is helpful to examine both the beat to beat interval plot (**Figure 25a**) and the marker channel strip (**Figure 25b**). The interval plot illustrates an abrupt change in heart rate [1] following a period of stable heart rates with gradual variations.

Pacing Summary

Mode		Rates	
Mode	AAI<=>DDD	Lower	55 bpm
Mode Switch	171 bpm	Upper Track	140 bpm
		Upper Sensor	140 bpm

AV Intervals		Additional Features	
Paced AV	270 ms	Rate Drop Response	On
Sensed AV	270 ms	Detection Type	Drop
		Drop Size	→ 25 bpm
		Drop Rate	→ 60 bpm
		Detection Window	1 min
		Intervention Rate	100 bpm
		Intervention Duration	2 min

Figure 25c.

2. The rate drop detection is defined by the three programmable parameters (**Figure 25c**), Drop Size, Drop Rate, and Detection Window. Detection is met if the ventricular rate drops below the Drop Rate by the Drop Size within the Detection Window. The marker channel strip in Figure 25b illustrates the detailed timing intervals. At first, the rate slows [2] from 110 bpm to 76 bpm. This meets the Drop Size (25 bpm), but does not meet the Drop Rate criteria (60 bpm) currently programmed for this patient.

3. This is followed by a significant drop in rate [3] with atrial pacing at the programmed lower rate of 55 bpm (1090 ms). Rate drop detection is met exceeding the Drop Size of 25 bpm and slowing below the Drop Rate of 60 bpm.

4. After detection is met, the device paces at the Intervention Rate of 100 bpm for the Intervention Duration defined by programmable parameters (Figure 25c). The device will incrementally step down the rate by 5 bpm every minute until it returns to the programmed lower rate of 55 bpm.

CLINICAL RESPONSE

Routine remote follow-up reports approximately 1300 rate drop episodes per month. Since pacemaker implantation with the Drop Rate feature programmed on, the patient's pre-syncope and syncope has resolved. It is crucial to combine pacing intervention with conservative therapy that includes liberal hydration, salt intake, and use of compression stockings in patients with cardioinhibitory neurocardiogenic syncope.

26 | Rate Smoothing

DEVICE: Boston Scientific Essentio EL L121 DC PM

PATIENT: A 62-year-old patient with paroxysmal atrial flutter experiences dizzy spells and rapid heart rates. The patient was in the ECG lab undergoing a 12-lead ECG. During the ECG measurement, runs of atrial flutter were observed, followed by asystole for 2- to 4-second intervals. The patient was referred to electrophysiology for consultation. Holter monitoring recorded ventricular rates up to 160 bpm and a 6.7-second pause as shown in **Figure 26a**. The patient underwent dual-chamber pacemaker placement and was started on metoprolol. Consider the following presenting EGM in **Figure 26b**.

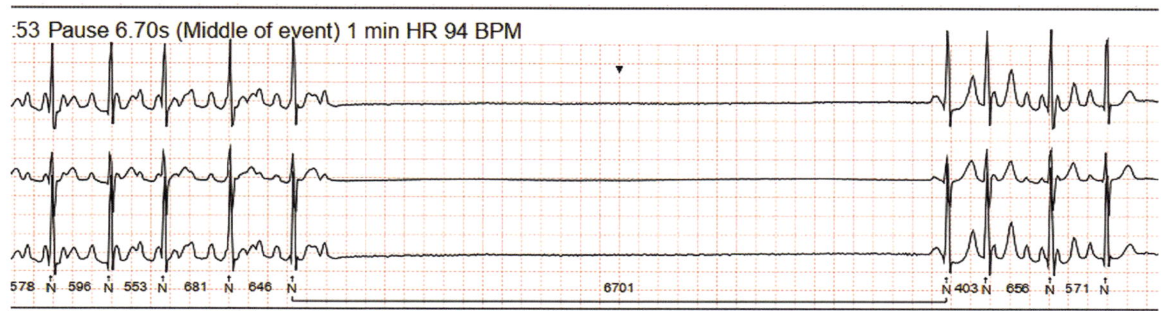

Figure 26a.

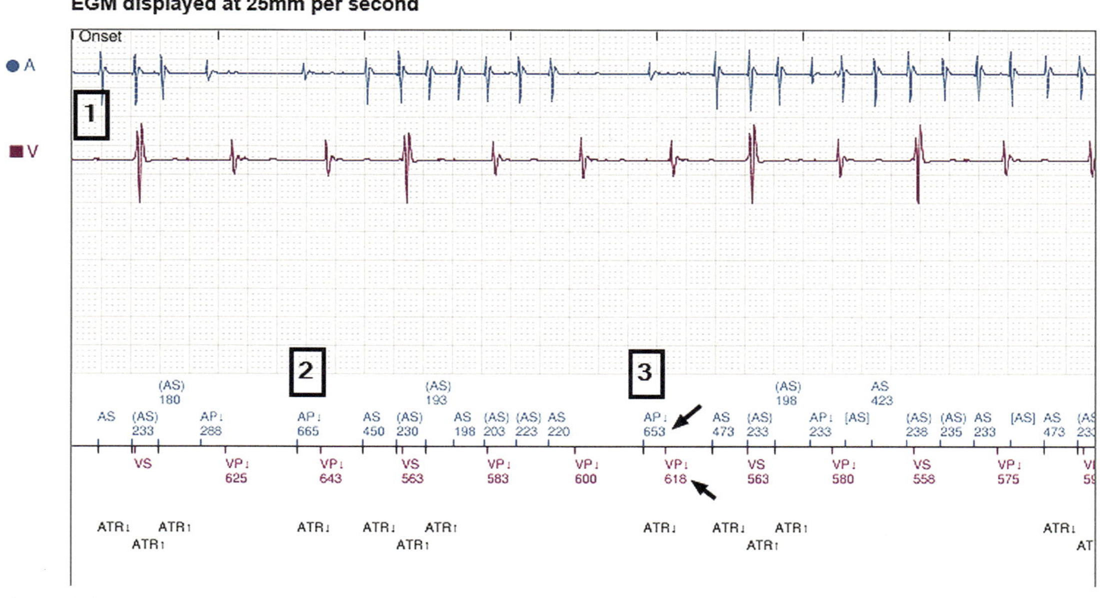

Figure 26b.

1. The presenting EGM in Figure 26b. is from routine remote follow-up and shows the patient's paroxysmal atrial flutter in progress. While the atrial flutter starts and stops, the ventricular rate has very little variation [1]. The Rate Smoothing feature is programmed on as shown in **Figure 26c**.

Settings		ATR Mode Switch Details	
Mode	DDDR	ATR Mode Switch	On
Lower Rate Limit	60 ppm	Trigger Rate	140 bpm
Maximum Tracking Rate	130 ppm	Duration	8 cycles
Maximum Sensor Rate	130 ppm	Entry Count	8 cycles
Paced AV Delay	110 - 250 ms	Exit Count	8 cycles
Sensed AV Delay	110 - 250 ms	Fallback	
A-Refractory (PVARP)	240 - 280 ms	Mode	DDIR
		Time	00:30 mm:ss
		ATR Fallback LRL	60 ppm

Rate Enhancements	
Rate Smoothing	
Up	Off
Down	3 %
Sudden Brady Response	Off

Figure 26c.

2. Rate Smoothing feature responds to atrial and/or ventricular rate fluctuations. It is indicated by the channel markers AP↓ and VP↓. Rate Smoothing is an enhancement to ATR Mode Switch and reduces the rate fluctuations associated with the onset and ending of atrial arrhythmias. In this case Rate Smoothing Down is programmed on and controls the largest pacing rate decrease allowed. The longest ventricular interval is defined by the previous R-to-R interval + 3%. The longest atrial interval is defined by previous R-to-R interval + 3% − AV Delay.

3. In this case the calculated ventricular paced Rate Smoothing interval [3] is 600 ms + 18 ms = 618 ms. The atrial paced interval [3] is earlier by the rate responsive AV delay of approximately 180 ms.

CLINICAL RESPONSE

The dual-chamber pacemaker eliminates pauses that occur during the patient's paroxysmal atrial fibrillation. The Rate Smoothing enhancement further eliminates fluctuation between atrial flutter rates and the programmed lower rate. The basic premise to minimize ventricular rate variation and perceived symptoms.

27 | Atrial Flutter Response

DEVICE: Boston Scientific Ingenio K173 DC PM

PATIENT: An active 83-year-old patient with a history of bradycardia and paroxysmal atrial flutter has a dual-chamber pacemaker. The patient exercises regularly using a rowing machine, indoor bike, or elliptical machine. Consider the following atrial tachycardia episode EGM from routine remote monitoring. What feature allows the device to mode switch?

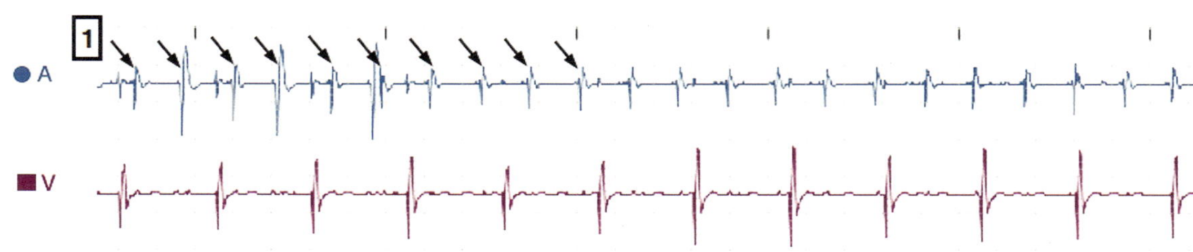

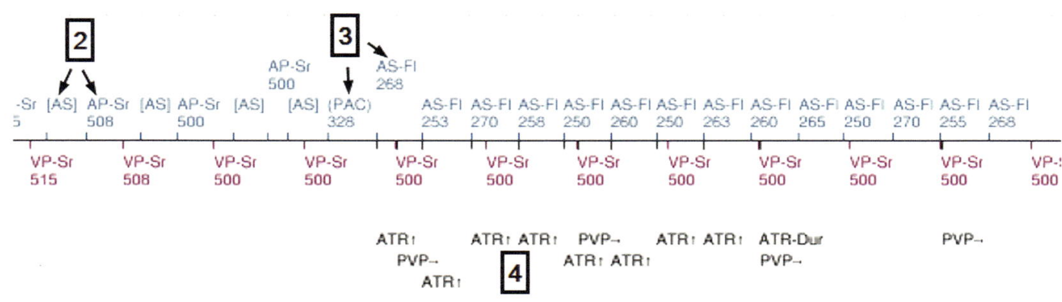

Figure 27a.

Settings

Mode	DDDR
RYTHMIQ™	Off
Lower Rate Limit	60 ppm
Maximum Tracking Rate	120 ppm
Maximum Sensor Rate	120 ppm
Paced AV Delay	200 - 200 ms
Sensed AV Delay	200 - 200 ms
A-Refractory (PVARP)	220 - 250 ms

Blanking

A-Blank after V-Pace	(125 ms)
A-Blank after V-Sense	45 ms
V-Blank after A-Pace	65 ms

Figure 27b.

ANALYSIS

1. The atrial EGM tracing shows consistent atrial flutter at a rate of approximately 214 bpm indicated by the arrows [1] in **Figure 27a**. At the beginning of the EGM, the atrial flutter waves are obscured (fused) with the pacing artifact.

2. At first, the device markers show atrial flutter waves are sensed in atrial blanking indicated by the [AS] marker (A-Blank after V-Pace = 125 ms). The device ignores the blanked atrial events [AS], and is dual-chamber pacing AP VP at the sensor indicated rate of 118 bpm (508 ms) with a paced AV delay of 200 ms as programmed (**Figure 27b**). The atrial pacing does capture the atrium as pacing occurs in the refractory period. The device does not recognize the atrial flutter. The VP events at the sensor reset the atrial blanking period (125 ms) allowing the pattern to repeat. The patient confirmed he was exercising at this time.

ATR Mode Switch Details

ATR Mode Switch	On
Trigger Rate	170 bpm
Duration	8 cycles
Entry Count	8 cycles
Exit Count	8 cycles
Fallback	
Mode	DDIR
Atrial Tachy Response	
Atrial Flutter Response	On
Trigger Rate	170 bpm
PMT Termination	On

Figure 27c.

3. The Atrial Flutter Response (AFR) feature is programmed on, as shown in **Figure 27c**. The AFR feature allows the device to detect atrial events in an AFR window independent of VP events. The AFR window is defined by the AFR trigger rate (60,000/170 bpm = 353 ms). It prevents atrial pacing into the vulnerable period and prevents tracking of high atrial rates. The atrial flutter event sensed in refractory [3] starts the AFR window. An atrial event detected in the AFR window is classified as a "sense" indicated by the AS-Fl marker and begins a new AFR window. Ventricular pacing is not affected by AFR and will take place as scheduled similar to VDIR mode.

4. Atrial events (AS-Fl) are now all counted toward ATR mode switch. Effectively, the atrial blanking is suspended and allows the device to appropriately mode switch.

CLINICAL RESPONSE

In this case, AFR is successfully functioning as designed and no changes were required.

28 | Atrial Tachyarrhythmia with Atrial Intervention Pacing

DEVICE: Medtronic Advisa DR MRI A2DR01 DC PM

PATIENT: A 76-year-old patient with a history of atrial flutter who underwent a pulmonary vein isolation ablation procedure experiences several episodes of syncope. During hospitalization a syncopal episode occurred and correlated with a 7-second sinus pause at atrial flutter conversion. The patient was subsequently implanted with a dual-chamber pacemaker with atrial tachyarrhythmia therapy capability given her history of atrial tachyarrhythmias.

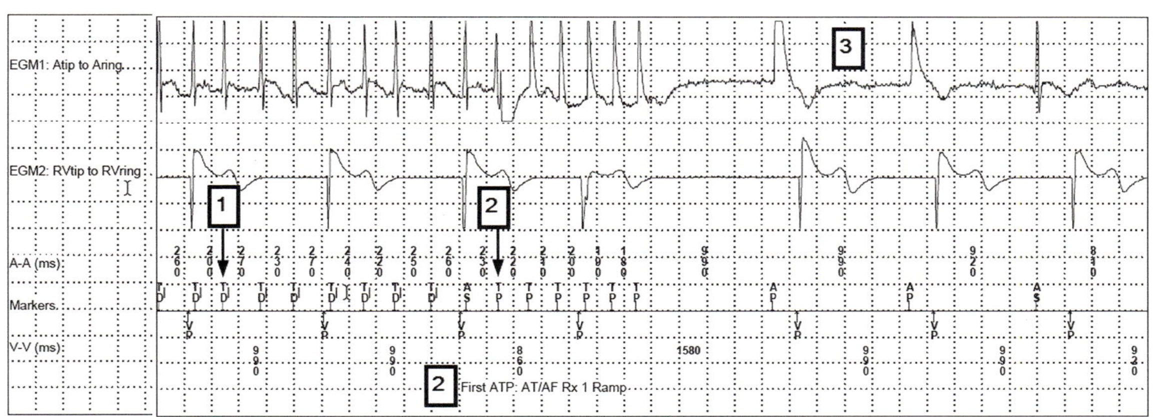

Figure 28a.

Parameter Summary

Mode	AAIR<=>DDDR	Lower Rate	60 bpm	Paced AV	180 ms
Mode Switch	150 bpm	Upper Track	130 bpm	Sensed AV	150 ms
		Upper Sensor	130 bpm		

Detection		Rates	Therapies
AT/AF	On (1 zone)	>150 bpm	Burst+, Ramp
VT	Monitor	>150 bpm	

Figure 28b.

ANALYSIS

1. Ventricular arrhythmia detection and therapy is the mainstay of ICD function. Atrial tachyarrhythmia detection and therapy is a less common function for an ICD. Medtronic offers this feature in select dual-chamber pacemaker and ICD models. The beginning of the EGM in **Figure 28a** shows a high atrial rate, likely to be atrial flutter. The TD marker [1] indicates an atrial tachyarrhythmia episode that has been detected.

2. The TP marker [2] indicates the atrial antitachycardia pacing (ATP) therapy is being delivered. The therapy is also indicated in the lower EGM notation [2]. In this example, the atrial ATP sequence sequence (6 consecutive beats, RAMP) was successful and terminated the atrial tachyarrhythmia [3].

CLINICAL RESPONSE

It is easy to overlook the fact that atrial therapies are programmed on [4] as shown in **Figure 28b**. When implanting a device equipped with atrial intervention pacing, it is recommended not to program AT/AF therapy 'on' until the atrial lead has matured. If a newly implanted atrial lead dislodges into the ventricle, sensing may be arbitrary. This may result in inappropriate detection of an atrial rhythm and delivery of therapy (ATP or cardioversion) to the ventricle with the potential for inducing ventricular arrhythmia.

29 | Mode Switch Termination with Failure to Establish AV Synchrony

DEVICE: Boston Scientific Essentio L101 DC PM

PATIENT: An 86-year-old with hypertrophic cardiomyopathy patient with a history of paroxysmal atrial fibrillation receives a pacemaker for symptomatic sick sinus syndrome. Routine remote follow-up indicated atrial tachycardia events. The EGM tracing (**Figure 29a**) is obtained from routine remote follow-up.

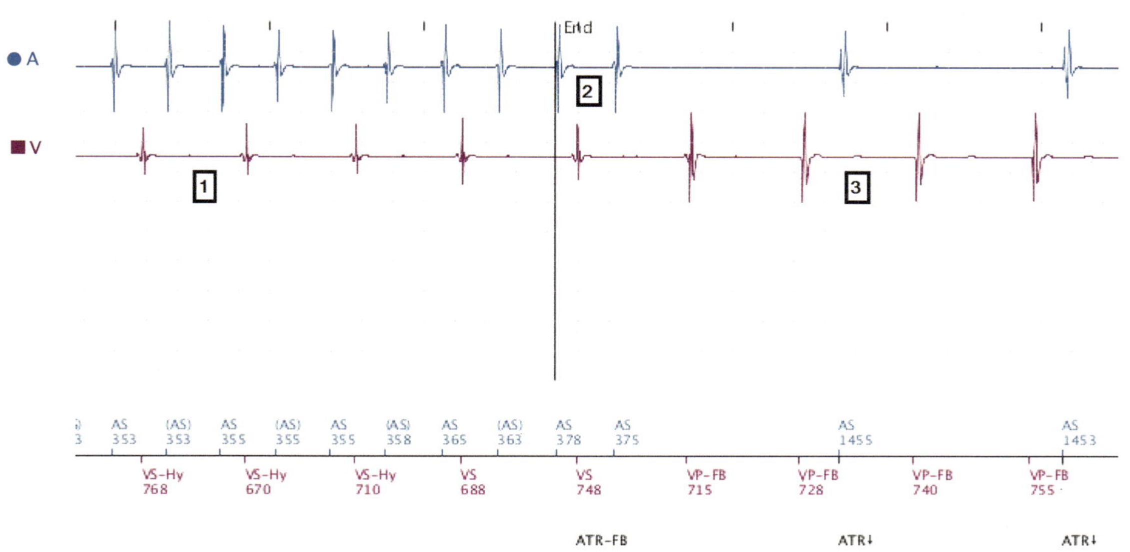

Figure 29a.

ATR Mode Switch Details

ATR Mode Switch	On
Trigger Rate	150 bpm
Duration	8 cycles
Entry Count	8 cycles
Exit Count	8 cycles
Fallback	
Mode	VDIR
Time	00:30 mm:ss
ATR Fallback LRL	60 ppm

Figure 29b.

1. Patient in mode switch for atrial flutter.

2. Mode switch ended.

3. The patient only had pacing in the ventricle given the patient's slow sinus rate due to mode switch being programmed to VDIR pacing mode. As noted in the programmed parameters in **Figure 29b**, the programmed mode-switch "mode" is VDIR. In this mode, the patient will maintain AV synchrony by tracking the atrial rate if the intrinsic atrial rate is greater than the programmed lower rate. If the sinus rate is slow, as in this patient, the VDIR mode effectively functions as VVIR until faster sinus rate is established. The ventricular pacing rate is around 80 bpm, which is likely the sensor-indicated rate at that time. In most patients, it is desirable to maintain AV synchrony to the greatest extent possible. As a result of this remote finding, the patient was scheduled to come into the clinic for follow-up and reprogramming of the mode switch from VDIR to DDIR.

30 | Inappropriate Mode Switch

DEVICE: St. Jude Medical* Assurity 2240 DC PM

PATIENT: This 80-year-old male was implanted with a dual-chamber pacemaker for paroxysmal atrial fibrillation and intermittent AV block. The tracing below was obtained from a routine remote transmission. Does this EGM show appropriate detection of an atrial arrhythmia?

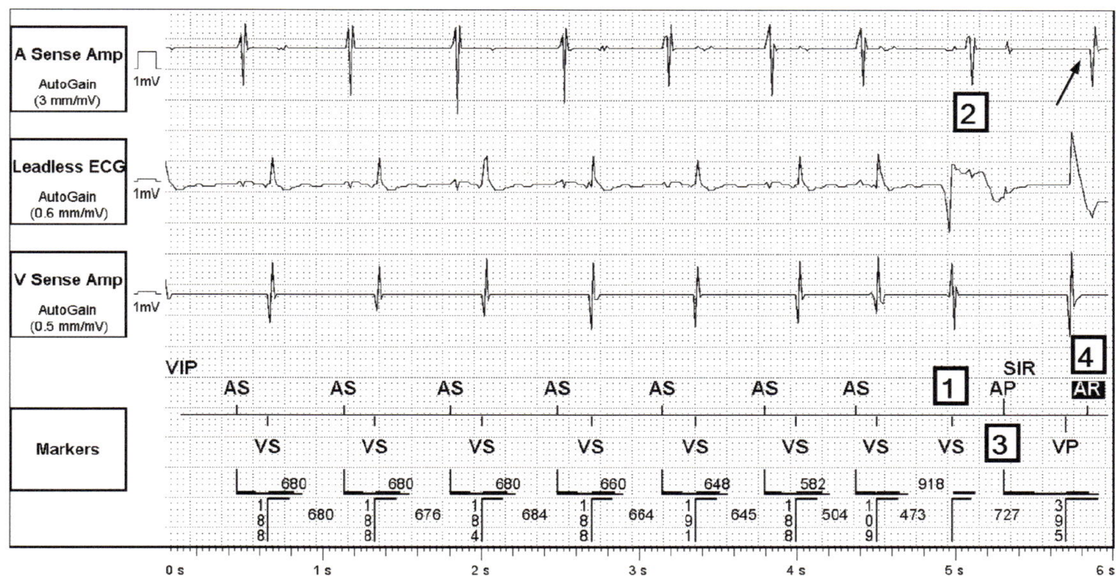

Figure 30a.

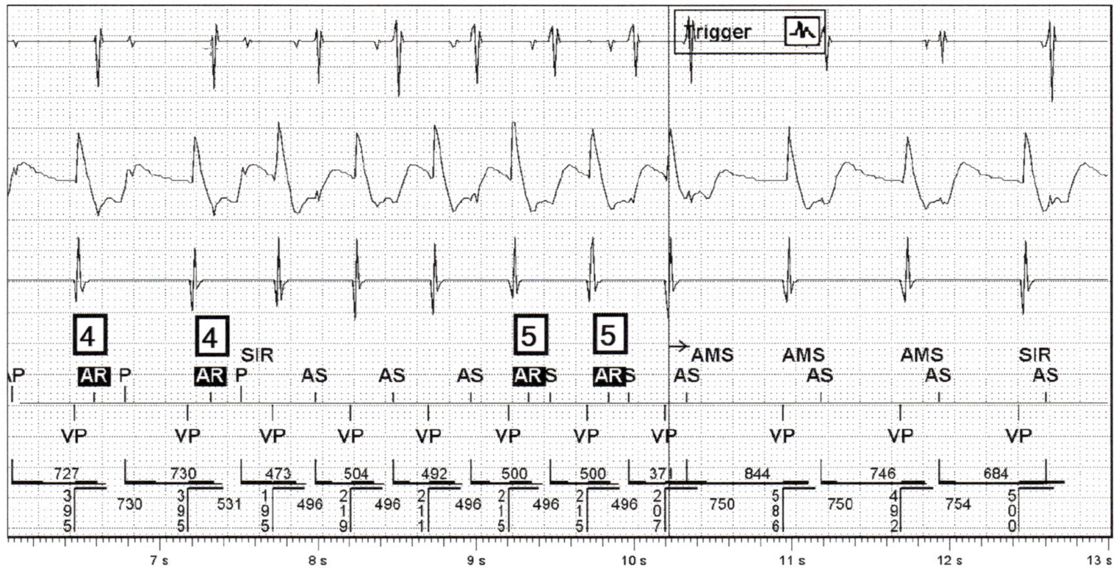

Figure 30b.

---

*St. Jude Medical is now Abbott.

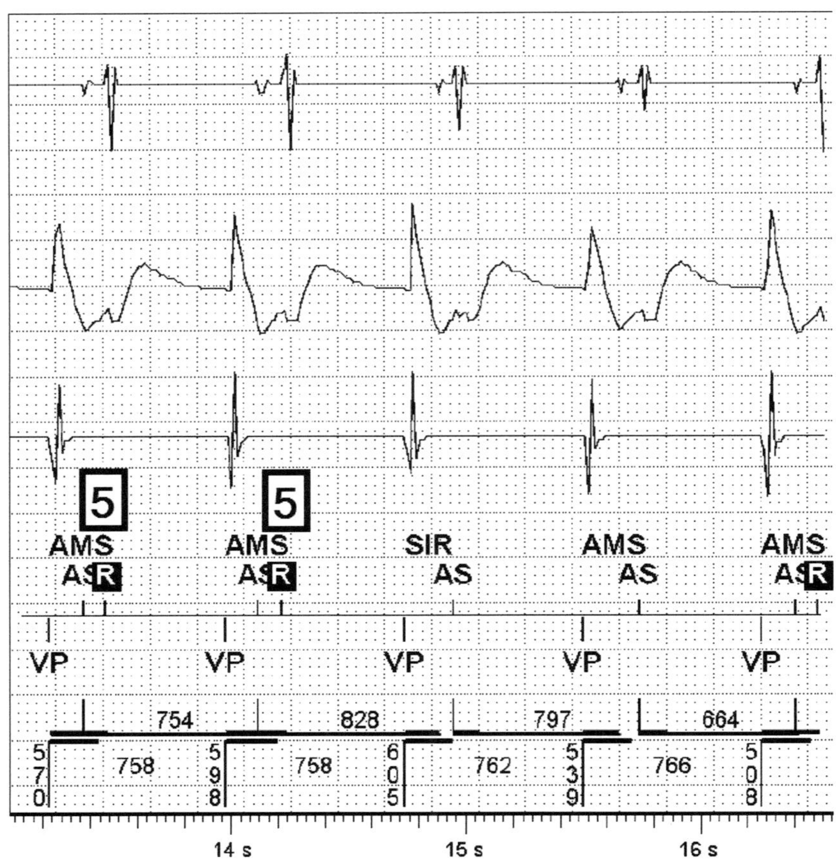

Figure 30c.

Basic Operation		**Refractories & Blanking**	
Mode	DDDR	PVARP	275 ms
		Post-Vent. Atrial Blanking	150 ms
Rates			
Base Rate	60 bpm	PVC Response	Atrial Pace
Delays		**AT/AF Detection & Response**	
Paced AV Delay	200 ms	Auto Mode Switch	DDIR
Sensed AV Delay	150 ms	A. Tachycardia Detection Rate	150 bpm
		AMS Base Rate	60 bpm

Capture & Sense	**A**	**V**
Sensitivity (Safety Margin)	0.5 mV (4.8:1)	Auto ❹

Delays			
Paced AV Delay	200 ms	Ventricular Intrinsic Preference (VIP®)	On
Sensed AV Delay	150 ms	VIP® Extension	200 ms
Rate Responsive AV Delay	Off	Search Interval	30 min
		Search Cycles	3

Figure 30d.

1. The EGM in **Figure 30a** shows sinus rhythm with a premature ventricular complex (PVC) [1].

2. The intrinsic sinus P wave [2] following the PVC falls within the postventricular atrial blanking period (PVABP).

3. The PVC response is programmed to Atrial Pace, therefore the pulse generator delivers an atrial pace 330 ms after the PVC. This paced impulse does not capture the atrium as it is still refractory (functional non-capture); therefore, after the paced AV delay of 200 ms, a ventricular pacing impulse is delivered.

4. The subsequent ventricular paced event places the P wave that follows [4] within the postventricular atrial refractory period (PVARP). This P wave appears to be of retrograde conduction, evidenced by the change in morphology (see arrow). The following two P waves are sinus in origin; however, due to these P waves falling into the PVARP [4], the device delivers a non-captured/non-conducted atrial pace shortly after each, i.e., functional non-capture.

5. Another contributing factor occurs with FFRW oversensing. The FFRW either falls into the PVARP and is denoted AR, followed, most likely, by retrograde VA conduction with AS notation (see [5] in **Figure 30b**) or, when the FFRW falls outside the PVARP and is denoted with AS markers, the next intrinsic sinus P wave falls into the Atrial refractory period and is denoted AR (see [5] in **Figure 30c**). Of note, in Figures 30a and 30b, the AV delay is extended to 400 ms due to a VIP extension of 200 ms. Following the third cycle with no ventricular sensed event occurring after the atrial events, the device returns to the programmed AV delay of 200 ms. The arrow in Figure 30b points to where this occurred.

6. Both phenomena led to an inappropriate AMS because, in this company's device, Atrial Sensed, Atrial Refractory, and Atrial Paced events count toward a Filtered Atrial Rate Interval (FARI) that exceeds the programmed Atrial Tachycardia Detection Rate (ATR) of 150 bpm as noted in the parameters (see **Figure 30d**). Normally, the device would revert to the programmed mode, i.e., exit AMS, when the FARI fell below the MTR or the Sensor Driven rate. However, in this example FFRW oversensing prevents this mode reversion, as seen in Figure 30c.

Atrial paced events continue to count toward Mode Switch. The FFRW oversensing can be eliminated by either extending PVAB and/or decreasing atrial sensitivity. The patient has consistent P wave measuring between 1.7 mV and 3.4 mV. Currently, the atrial sensitivity is set to 0.5 mV, giving him nearly a 5× safety margin. Adjusting the atrial sensitivity to 0.7 mV might address the FFRW oversensing without risk of undersensing atrial fibrillation.

31 | Loss of AV Synchrony Due to Inappropriate Mode Switch

DEVICE: Boston Scientific Energen N141 CRT-D

PATIENT: A 44-year-old female was implanted with a CRT-D device for management of heart failure secondary to cardiac sarcoidosis. The EGM from an ATR episode is shown below in **Figures 31a**, **31b**, and **31c** and the programmed settings are seen in **Figure 31d**.

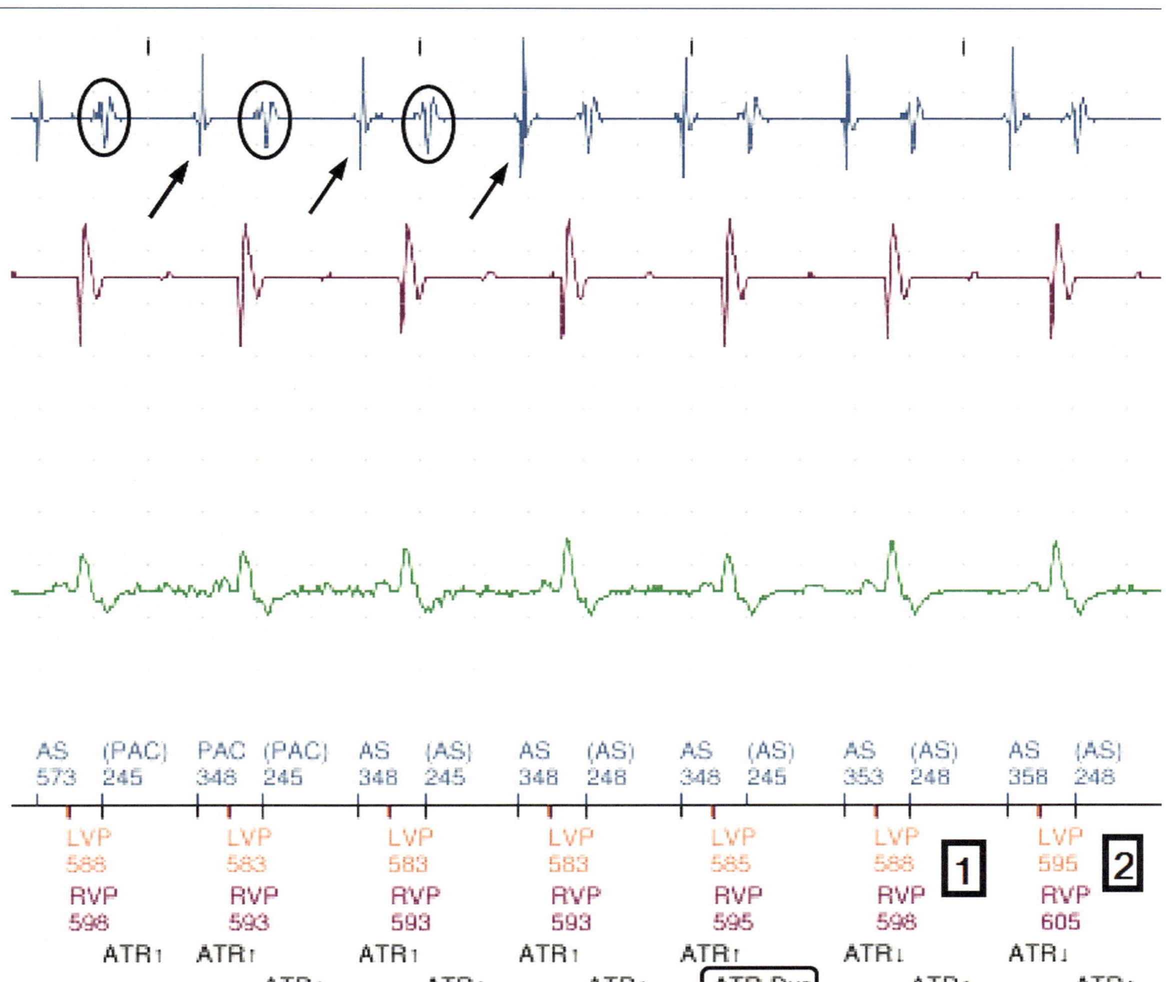

Figure 31a.

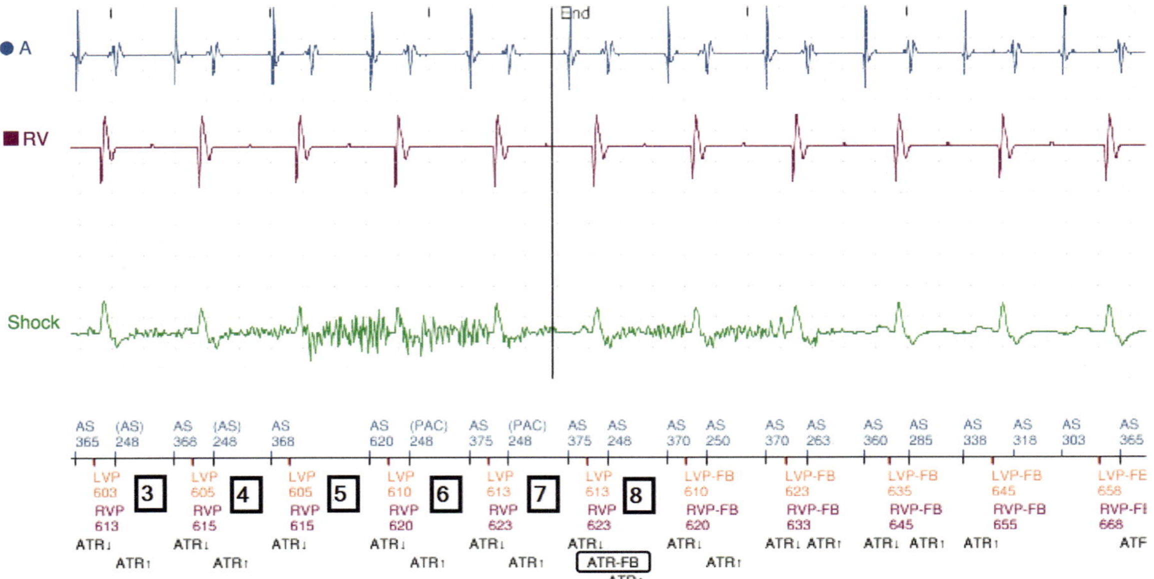

Figure 31b.

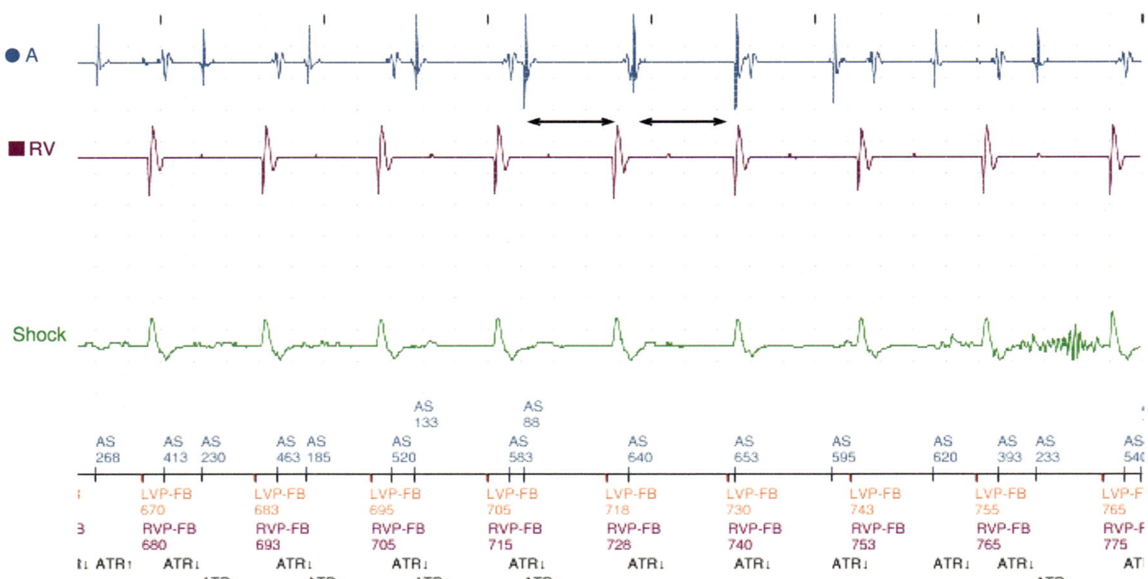

Figure 31c.

Normal Settings		Atrial Tachy	
Mode	DDD	**Therapy**	
Lower Rate Limit	50 ppm	**ATR Mode Switch Details**	
Maximum Tracking Rate	110 ppm	ATR Mode Switch	On
Paced AV Delay	120 - 120 ms	Trigger Rate	170 bpm
Sensed AV Delay	120 - 120 ms	Duration	8 cycles
A-Refractory (PVARP)	350 - 350 ms	Entry Count	8 cycles
RV-Refractory (RVRP)	250 - 250 ms	Exit Count	8 cycles
LV-Refractory (LVRP)	250 ms	Fallback	
Ventricular Pacing Chamber	BiV	Mode	VDI
LV Offset	-10 ms	Time	00:30 mm:ss
PVARP after PVC	400 ms	ATR/VTR Fallback LRL	60 ppm
LV Protection Period	350 ms	Ventricular Rate Regulation	Min
Blanking		BiV Trigger	On
A-Blank after V-Pace	Smart	Maximum Pacing Rate	110 ppm
A-Blank after RV-Sense	Smart		
RV-Blank after A-Pace	65 ms		
LV-Blank after A-Pace	65 ms		

Figure 31d.

ANALYSIS

1. In Figure 31a, oversensing of FFRWs on the atrial channel, identified by circles, in addition to the true sinus P waves, identified by arrows, both count toward the detection of an ATR; in combination, they occur at a rate faster than the ATR trigger rate of 170 bpm. There are alternating short/long intervals noted due to FFRW sensing followed by native P waves. True flutter waves would have a constant cycle length. Once the number of fast atrial events meets the ATR Entry count, in this case eight cycles, the device initiates a Duration count, denoted by ATR-Dur. Per the programmed settings seen in Figure 31d, in order for Duration to be met, the fast atrial events must persist for the next eight ventricular cycles. Each fast atrial event counts up toward Entry and, in this case, a maximum of eight. While each slow atrial event counts down from the maximum of eight toward the Exit count of zero. If the count reached zero before the next eight ventricular cycles, the device would exit the episode and no mode switch would occur.

2. In Figure 31b, after the eight ventricular cycles occur without the Exit count reaching zero, a Mode Switch is triggered, denoted by ATR-FB, and the Mode changes to a nontracking mode, in this case VDI mode.

3. In Figure 31c, due to this inappropriate mode switch and the nontracking mode of VDI, there is AV dissociation. The FFRWs can be easily recognized from native P waves after AV dissociation.

CLINICAL RESPONSE

The oversensing of FFRWs on the atrial channel can be eliminated by changing the A-Blank after V-pace from the SMART setting, which is 37.5 ms to 105 ms.

32 | Auto-PVARP and Inappropriate Mode Switch

DEVICE: Medtronic Azure XT DR MRI W1DR01 DC PM

PATIENT: A 48-year-old patient who developed complete heart block after mitral valve surgery received a dual-chamber pacemaker. Multiple AT/AF episodes are reported with routine remote monitoring. Consider the AT/AF episode and EGM shown in **Figure 32a** and **32c**. (Programmed settings are shown in **Figure 32b**.) A cursory look at the atrial EGM may lead you to agree with the device's classification of atrial tachyarrhythmia and appropriate mode switch.

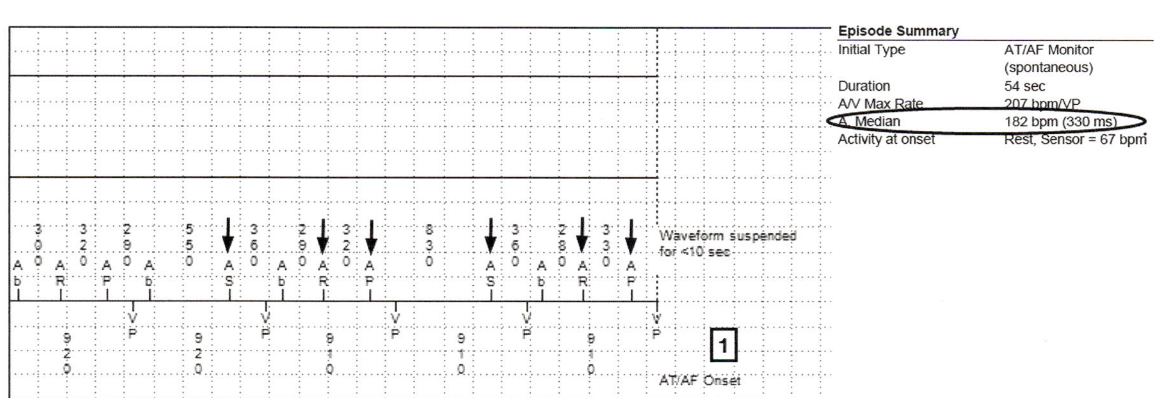

Figure 32a.

Pacing Summary

Mode		Rates		AV Intervals	
Mode	DDDR	Lower	60 bpm	Paced AV	180 ms
Mode Switch	171 bpm	Upper Track	145 bpm	Sensed AV	150 ms
		Upper Sensor	145 bpm		

AT/AF Detection

Detection	A. Interval (Rate)
Monitor	
AT/AF	350 ms (171 bpm)

Refractory/Blanking

PVARP	Auto
Minimum PVARP	250 ms

Additional Features

Non-Comp Atrial Pacing	On
NCAP Interval	300 ms

Figure 32b.

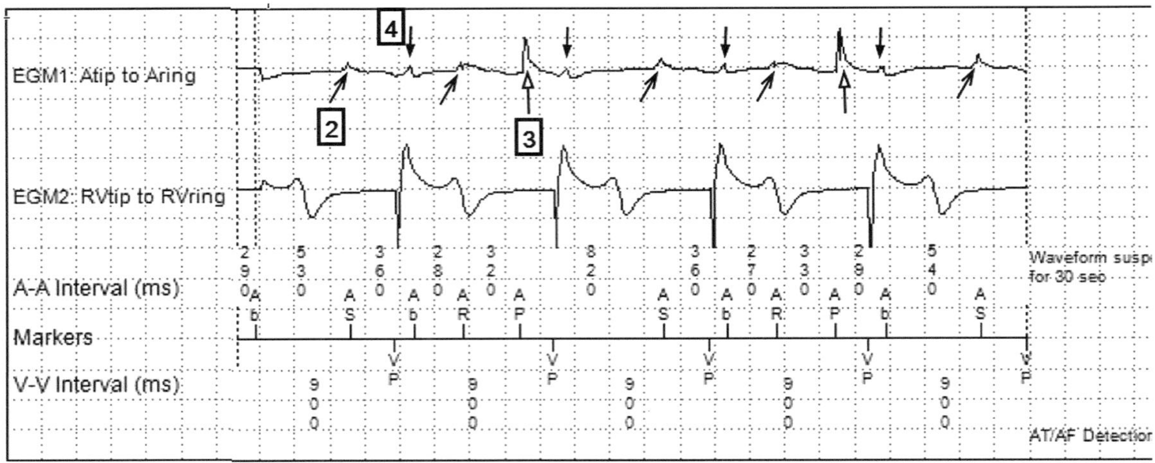

Figure 32c.

ANALYSIS

1. In Figure 32a the device identifies AT/AF onset [1] when the median of the 12 most recent atrial intervals is shorter than the programmed AT/AF detection. In this episode the median atrial cycle length was 330 ms, less than programmed AT/AF detection of 350 ms (Figure 32b). The atrial events identified by markers AS, AR, or AP are counted as AT/AF intervals. The intervals that fall into postventricular atrial blanking (PVAB), intervals marked Ab, are not counted.

2. Careful inspection of the EGM waveforms in Figure 32c reveals three distinct categories of atrial events. Atrial events [2] with markers AS or AR correspond to intrinsic atrial activity. This intrinsic rhythm is likely sinus rhythm with bigeminal PACs. The intrinsic PAC events fall into postventricular atrial refractory period (PVARP), marked AR, as a result of the Auto PVARP feature (Figure 32b). Auto PVARP varies the length of PVARP based on the current pacing rate. It lengthens PVARP at slower rates to promote AV synchrony and avoid PMT; it shortens PVARP at faster rates to prevent atrial competitive pacing. Auto PVARP attempts to maintain a 300-ms window between the end of PVARP and the next atrial pace (PVARP = Sensor rate interval – Paced AV – 300 ms). PVARP = ~1000 ms – 180 ms – 300 ms = 520 ms. The PAC events occur 400 ms after the ventricular pace and therefore fall into PVARP.

3. The timing of the AP paced events [3] following an AR result from lower rate timing or from the non-competitive atrial pacing (NCAP) interval. The NCAP feature prevents pacing the atrium within the vulnerable period of the atrium. If the atrial pace is schedule to occur during the NCAP interval, the atrial pace is delayed and the paced AV interval is decreased. In this case, the rate responsive lower rate of 960 ms (360 + 280 + 320 ms) determines the AS to AP interval and NCAP = 300 ms is not violated. The AR events resulting from the extended PVARP are ignored by the atrial timer but included in the AT/AF counters. The combination of the AR events followed by the unnecessary atrial paced event adds inappropriately to the AT/AF counters resulting in the inappropriate AT/AF detection.

4. Atrial events [4] correspond with each ventricular paced event and are assigned marker Ab. These atrial events are far-field artifact on the atrial EGM as a result of the ventricular paced events. These events fall into PVAB and are appropriately blanked from atrial counters.

CLINICAL RESPONSE

In this case, Auto PVARP resulted in inappropriate identification of AT/AF events. The events and timings were reviewed with Medtronic technical support. The recommendation was to turn off Auto PVARP and program a fixed PVARP of 250 ms. This resulted in appropriate tracking of the intrinsic atrial rhythm.

33 | Pacemaker-Mediated Tachycardia

DEVICE: Medtronic Sensia SEDR01 DC PM

PATIENT: An 86-year-old patient with a history of paroxysmal atrial flutter and high-grade AV block received a dual-chamber pacemaker. The patient was having a routine, annual ECG performed when a sudden change in paced rate was noted (**Figure 33a**). A subsequent EGM is shown in **Figure 33b**. What is the etiology of the more rapidly paced rhythm that was captured on the ECG?

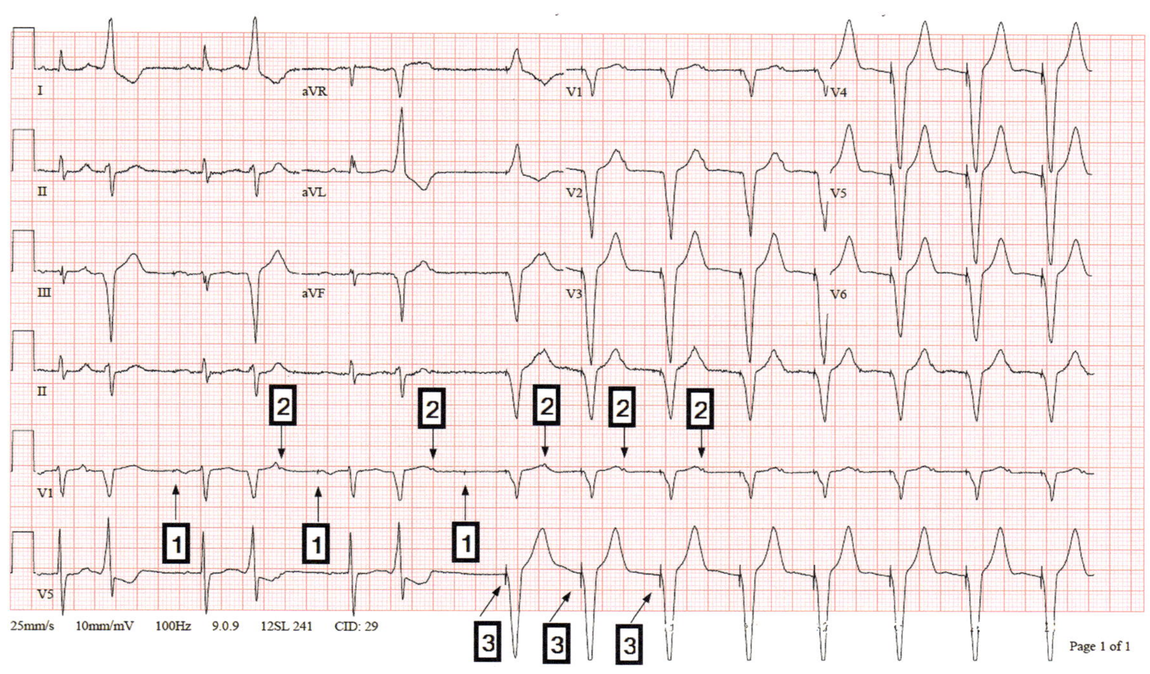

Figure 33a.

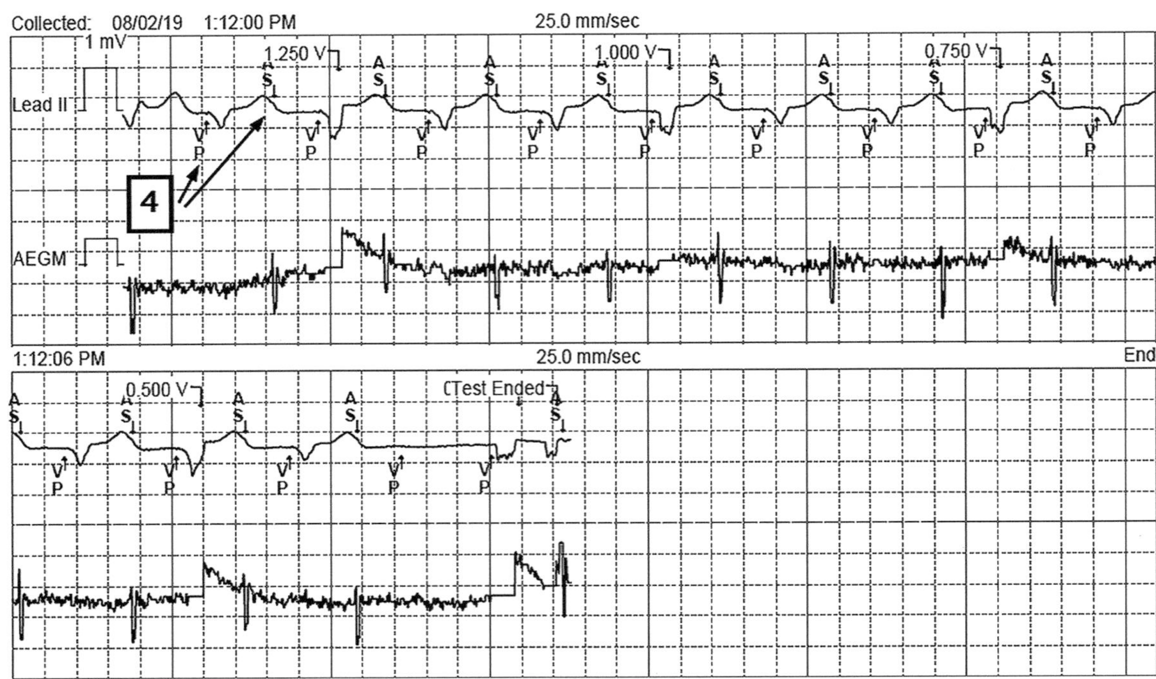

Figure 33b.

Modes

Mode	DDDR
Mode Switch	On
Detection Rate	175 bpm
Detection Duration	No Delay
Blanked Flutter Search	On

Rates

Lower Rate	50 ppm
Upper Tracking Rate	140 ppm
Upper Sensor Rate	140 ppm
ADL Rate	95 ppm

Intrinsic/AV

Paced AV	270 ms
Sensed AV	270 ms
Search AV+	On
Max Increase to AV	170 ms
Rate Adaptive AV	Off

Refractory/Blanking

PVARP	Auto
Minimum PVARP	250 ms
PVAB	180 ms
Ventricular Refractory	230 ms
Vent. Blanking (after A. Pace)	28 ms
PMT Intervention	On
PVC Response	On
Ventricular Safety Pacing	On

Figure 33c.

1. In Figure 33a, the ECG shows atrial pacing at a rate of 50 bpm. PVCs were noted following the first three atrial pacing events. However, on the third [1] atrial impulse, we see functional loss of capture. This may have resulted from the P wave falling in a refractory period following atrial activation conducted retrogradely after a PVC.

2. In Figure 33a, the ECG demonstrates retrograde atrial events following two PVCs and labeled with the first and second [2↓] The retrograde atrial events fall in the post-ventricular atrial refractory period (PVARP). On the third, fourth, and fifth complexes that are labeled with [2↓], we see the retrograde atrial event is tracked, i.e., associated with ventricular pacing [3].

3. As shown in **Figure 33c**, the device was programmed to DDD with a lower rate at 50 bpm.

4. The patient was seen in the clinic for pacemaker interrogation and testing. Figure 33b illustrates retrograde V-A conduction when the patient is paced in the ventricle.

CLINICAL RESPONSE

The patient was seen in the clinic for a pacemaker interrogation and reprogramming of the device. The interrogation showed that in a six-month window, the patient paced 20% in the atrium and 1% in the ventricle. An atrial threshold was determined and revealed a threshold of 0.5 V at 0.4 ms and the programmed device atrial amplitude was 1.5 V at 0.4 ms. No atrial loss of capture was noted during the interrogation. The patient was paced VVI at 90 bpm, and it was noted that the patient had V-to-A retrograde conduction with a timing cycle of 440 ms. The patient was asymptomatic with this testing. As a result of these findings, auto PVARP was turned off and a fixed PVARP was programmed to 460 ms. The paced AV delay was programmed from 270 ms to 200 ms, and the sensed AV delay was programmed from 270 ms to 200 ms. Upper tracking rate and the upper sensor rates were programmed from 140 bpm to 115 bpm. Rate adaptive AV delay was turned on to have a maximum AV delay of 140 ms. The search AV was programmed OFF. All of the following changes are illustrated in **Figure 33d**.

Any loss of AV synchrony may start pacemaker-mediated tachycardia in a patient with retrograde conduction. RV pacing avoidance algorithms promote long AV delays, which in turn may increase the chance of VA conduction with events like PVCs. In some patients, when the VA interval is too long, we may have to pace the ventricle with a shorter AV delay to avoid retrograde conduction.

Modes

	Initial	Final
Mode	DDDR	DDDR
Mode Switch	On	On
Detection Rate	175 bpm	175 bpm
Detection Duration	No Delay	No Delay
Blanked Flutter Search	On	On

Rates

Lower Rate	50 ppm		50 ppm
Upper Tracking Rate	140 ppm	>	115 ppm
Upper Sensor Rate	140 ppm	>	115 ppm
ADL Rate	95 ppm		95 ppm

Intrinsic/AV

Paced AV	270 ms	>	200 ms
Sensed AV	270 ms	>	200 ms
Search AV+	On	>	Off
Max Increase to AV	170 ms		
Rate Adaptive AV	Off	>	On
Start Rate			80 ppm
Stop Rate			120 ppm
Maximum Offset			-60 ms

Refractory/Blanking

PVARP	Auto	>	460 ms
Minimum PVARP	250 ms		
PVAB	180 ms		180 ms
Ventricular Refractory	230 ms		230 ms
Vent. Blanking (after A. Pace)	28 ms		28 ms
PMT Intervention	On		On
PVC Response	On		On
Ventricular Safety Pacing	On		On

Figure 33d.

34 | Pacemaker-Mediated Tachycardia Intervention

DEVICE: Boston Scientific Essentio EL L121 DC PM

PATIENT: An 88-year-old patient received a dual-chamber pacemaker for 2:1 AV block and bifascicular bundle branch block. Pacemaker-mediated tachycardia (PMT) episodes were reported in the patient's routine remote follow-up. PMT occurs when the device tracks retrograde conducted P waves that fall out of the refractory period. The EGM from the PMT episode is shown in **Figure 34a** below. **Figure 34b** shows programmed pacing settings. Are retrograde P waves propagating PMT?

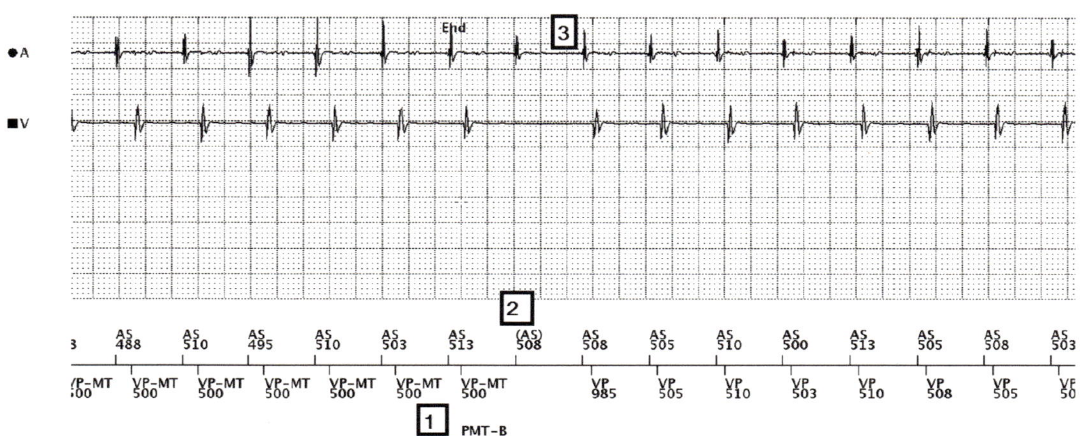

Figure 34a.

Settings

Mode	DDD
Lower Rate Limit	60 ppm
Maximum Tracking Rate	120 ppm
Maximum Sensor Rate	120 ppm
Paced AV Delay	80 - 180 ms
Sensed AV Delay	65 - 150 ms
A-Refractory (PVARP)	240 - 280 ms

Figure 34b.

ANALYSIS

1. The device has detected atrial tracking at the programmed MTR and classifies this episode as PMT. This is indicated by the ventricular pacing–maximum tracking (VP–MT) markers [1]. The device also labels the EGM with PMT-B. The maximum tracking interval of 500 ms corresponds to the programmed MTR of 120 bpm, Figure 34b. This device features a PMT detection and intervention algorithm. PMT is detected after 16 successive V-to-A intervals are counted at the MTR with less than 32 ms of V-to-A variation.

2. When the PMT condition is met (PMT-B marker), the device intervenes by extending the postventricular atrial blanking period (PVABP) to 500 ms for one cycle in order to prevent tracking in an attempt to break the PMT. The subsequent atrial event falls into the 500 ms refractory period, as indicated by the (AS) on the marker channel [2]. This atrial event is not tracked by the device.

3. The next waveform is another atrial sensed event [3] in the absence of ventricular pacing, confirming the atrial rhythm is not the result of retrograde conduction. The pattern continues with ventricular tracking of atrial sensed events. Unfortunately, the stored EGM does not show the initiation of the episode. The most likely conclusion is appropriate ventricular tracking of an intrinsic atrial rate that approximates the MTR of 120 bpm.

CLINICAL RESPONSE

Patient follow-up was conducted by phone. The patient did not recall any symptoms around the time of this episode. The patient's rate histogram diagnostic data did not indicate any significant or sustained tachycardia. This was an isolated event, no programming changes were made. The patient continues with routine remote monitoring.

35 | Pacemaker-Mediated Tachycardia in CRT-P

DEVICE: Boston Scientific Valitude X4 U128 CRT-P

PATIENT: An 80-year-old patient received a CRT-P for episodic bifasicular block following transfemoral aortic valve replacement. The patient also has nonischemic cardiomyopathy and left bundle branch block with QRS duration >150 ms. Holter monitoring demonstrates a PVC burden of 20%. Routine remote follow-up reports multiple PMT episodes. A typical PMT episode is shown in **Figure 35a**. Parameters are shown in **Figure 35b**. What programming options should be considered?

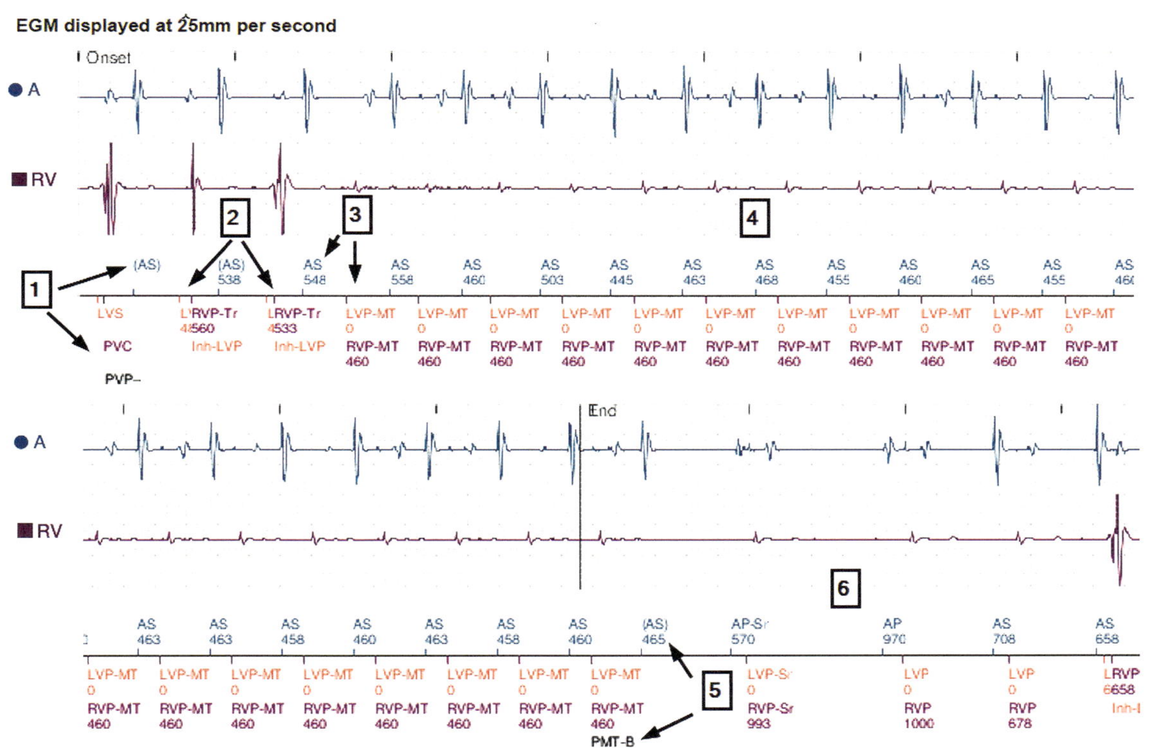

Figure 35a.

Settings

Mode	DDDR
Lower Rate Limit	60 ppm
Maximum Tracking Rate	130 ppm
Maximum Sensor Rate	130 ppm
Paced AV Delay	130 - 130 ms
Sensed AV Delay	100 - 100 ms
A-Refractory (PVARP)	280 - 320 ms
RV-Refractory (RVRP)	230 - 250 ms
LV-Refractory (LVRP)	250 ms
Ventricular Pacing Chamber	BiV
LV Offset	0 ms
PVARP after PVC	400 ms
LV Protection Period	400 ms

Output

●A	2.2 V @ 0.4 ms
■RV	Auto 2.0 V @ 0.4 ms
◆LV	1.5 V @ 0.4 ms

Sensitivity

●A	Fixed 1.0 mV
■RV	Fixed 2.5 mV
◆LV	Fixed 2.5 mV

ATR Mode Switch Details

ATR Mode Switch	On
Trigger Rate	170 bpm
Duration	8 cycles
Entry Count	8 cycles
Exit Count	8 cycles
Fallback	
Mode	DDIR
Time	00:30 mm:ss
ATR Fallback LRL	60 ppm
Ventricular Rate Regulation	Min
BiV Trigger	On
Maximum Pacing Rate	130 ppm

Atrial Tachy Response

Atrial Flutter Response	On
Trigger Rate	170 bpm
PMT Termination	On

Ventricular Regulation

BiV Trigger	On

Rate Enhancements

Rate Smoothing	
Up	Off %
Down	Off %
Tracking Preference	On
Sudden Brady Response	Off

Figure 35b.

ANALYSIS

1. The PVP→ channel marker [1] indicates the PVARP after PVC (400 ms) timing feature. This is initiated by an RV sensed event without a preceding atrial sensed event. This is designed to prevent PMT due to retrograde conduction. Retrograde conduction with atrial sensing in refractory indicated by (AS) does appear to follow the ventricular event, LVS. In this case, the PVARP extension to 400 ms was not necessary, the programmed PVARP of 320 ms would have been sufficient.

2. The pattern of ventricular sensing of PVCs followed by atrial sensing continues for 2 cycles [2]. BiV trigger is programmed on; the device will attempt to trigger pace the RV and LV in order to maximize CRT pacing. The RV triggered pacing marker, RVP-Tr, is superimposed over the LVS marker. The Inh-LVP marker results from the PVC being sensed by the LV lead first, thus LV trigger pacing is withheld in order to prevent an LV pacing stimulus during the LV vulnerable period. The LV protection period (400 ms), disallows LV pacing after any LV sensed or paced event.

3. The retrograde AS following the third PVC [3] is not refractory because the Tracking Preference feature is programmed on. With tracking preference, if two successive cycles of an RV event is preceded by atrial sensed event in PVARP, the device shortens PVARP to allow tracking. Tracking preference is designed to support CRT delivery for atrial rates near, but below the MTR. This atrial sensed event [3] is tracked, LV and RV paced at the MTR of 130 bpm (460 ms). The sensed AV delay of 100 ms is extended; the device will not violate the maximum tracking interval of 460 ms.

4. In this case, this feature essentially disables PVARP after PVC, and allows tracking of the retrograde atrial event, and PMT ensues [4].

5. The PMT detection algorithm detects the PMT indicated by the marker PMT-B [5]. PMT detection is defined as 16 successive cycles of ventricular pacing following atrial sensing at the max tracking interval with V-to-A variation less than 32 ms. The PMT intervention is extension of PVARP to 500 ms for one cardiac cycle. The final retrograde atrial event [5] falls into refractory (AS) and is not tracked.

6. The PMT cycle is broken and the device follows programmed timing parameters.

CLINICAL RESPONSE

For this patient the combination of PVC activity and the Tracking Preference feature results in frequent PMT events. Tracking preference is nominally programmed on and is useful to maintain CRT pacing in patients during faster atrial rates. Tracking preference was programmed OFF. The frequent PVCs in this patient also impacted optimal BiV pacing percentage. Alternative antiarrhythmic control of the PVCs is being trialed for this patient; if antiarrhythmic drug therapy is not successful, an ablation of the PVC focus (foci) will also be considered.

36 | Respiratory Trends and Atrial Oversensing

DEVICE: Boston Scientific Inogen X4 G148 CRT-D

PATIENT: A 72-year-old male previously received a CRT-D device for nonischemic cardiomyopathy. Approximately one year later, he was admitted to the hospital for implant of a LVAD. The EGMs shown in **Figures 36a** and **36b** were obtained at the hospital bedside during his recovery from implant of the LVAD.

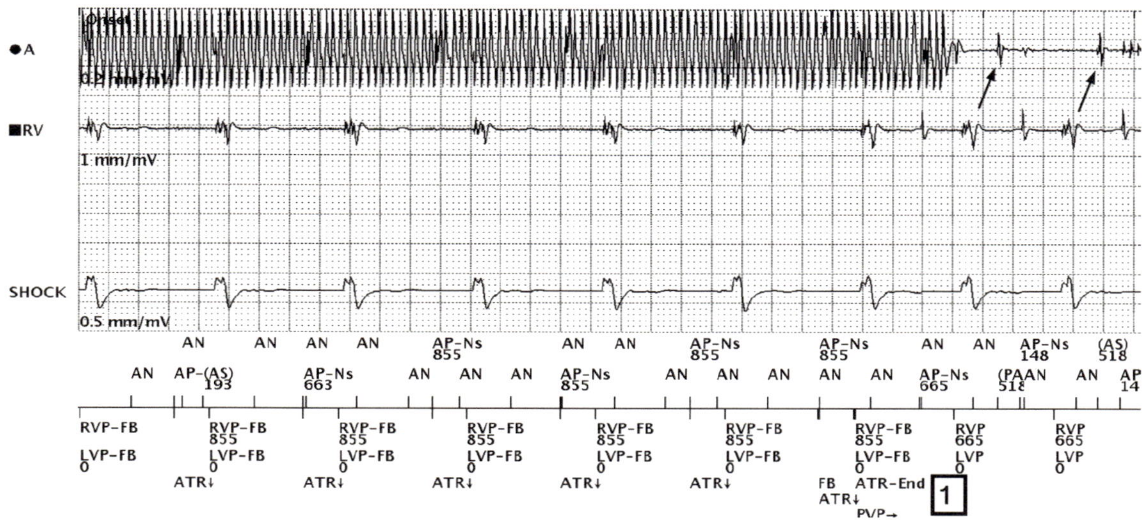

Figure 36a.

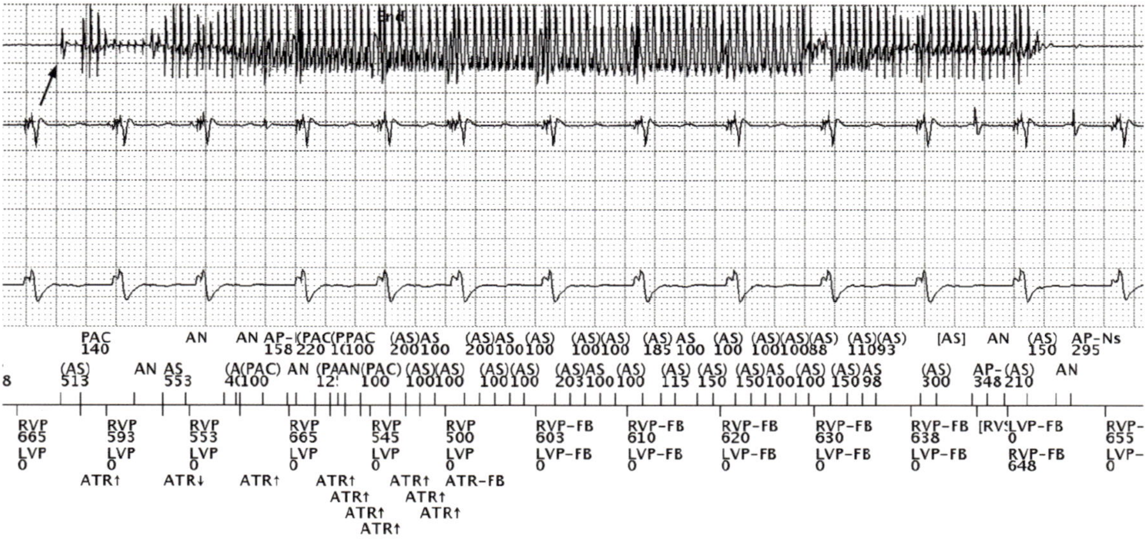

Figure 36b.

1. Both EGMs in Figures 36a and 36b are from the same episode, which the pulse generator inappropriately identifies as an ATR event. Ventricular pacing appropriately occurs at mode switch rate (VP-FB). The EGMs illustrate the phenomenon of atrial oversensing due to transthoracic impedance measurements (TIM). This issue is associated with Boston Scientific devices when Minute Ventilation or Respiratory Rate Trends are programmed as "on" in their pacemakers or CRT devices. This type oversensing has been observed[1] when the TIM occurs in a system that has high impedance within the ring circuit of the lead employed in TIM. The underlying mechanism is due to creation to creation of small particles due to lead material mismatch and subsequent oxidation leading to high impedance.[2] As constant current is applied during minute ventilation and with increased resistance (V=IR Ohm's law) increased voltage is applied on the lead. This increase voltage is sensed as the rapid signal by the device. Unfortunately, this oversensing has been known to produce pacing inhibition, inappropriate mode switching, and loss of AV synchrony and can be especially problematic for the pacemaker dependent patient.

2. While the same phenomenon is demonstrated in both EGMs, in the first EGM, the notation of 'AN' reflects that the device recognizes the signal as noise. Boston Scientific devices have a retriggerable noise rejection window and at the end of AV interval or VA a pacing impulse is delivered. In this patient atrial pacing continues throughout the period with noise. When the TIM oversensing stops briefly at the conclusion of the first EGM, the ATR episode ends. See [1] in Figure 36a. At this point in the episode, ventricular pacing produces retrograde conducted P waves (see arrows throughout). When the oversensing resumes in the second EGM, following the requisite eight ATR sensed events, the device inappropriately mode switches again. After a few seconds, the device recognized the noise once again and delivered atrial pacing impulses.

CLINICAL RESPONSE

For the pacemaker dependent patient, program Minute Ventilation and Respiratory Rate trends off. Consider using the components and of the CIED system that are from the same manufacturer. When minute ventilation is needed in a nonpacemaker-dependent patient, consider turning the signal artifact monitor "on" when such episodes are noted on the device.

1. Ryan JD, Tempel ND, Engle DD, et al. Oversensing of transthoracic excitation stimuli in contemporary pacemakers. *Pacing Clin Electrophysiol*. 2018;41:161–166. DOI: https://doi.org/10.1111/pace.13269

2. Tanawuttiwat T, Berger RD, Love CJ. Intermittent high impedance from the lead-device compatibility problem. *Heart Rhythm*. 2019;16(7):1107–1111. DOI: https://doi.org/10.1016/j.hrthm.2019.01.026

37 | Signal Artifact Monitor

DEVICE: Boston Scientific Essentio MRI EL L131 DC PM

PATIENT: An 80-year-old patient was implanted with a dual-chamber pacemaker for high-grade AV block with symptoms of fatigue and dyspnea. The patient also has a history of paroxysmal atrial fibrillation. The patient is in clinic for routine follow-up. Consider the following event with EGM listed in the arrhythmia logbook.

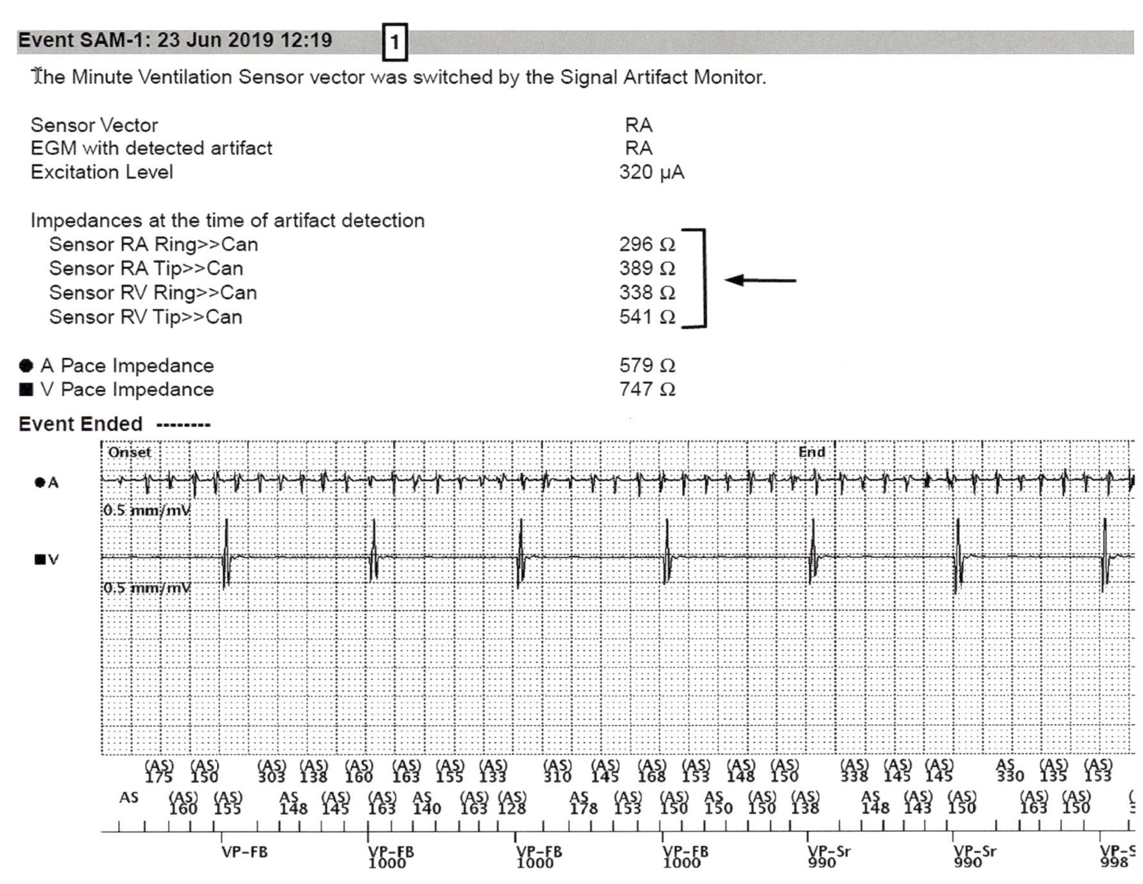

Figure 37a.

ANALYSIS

1. Signal Artifact Monitor (SAM) continuously monitors the EGMs for undesirable signal artifact that results from transthoracic impedance measurements. The Minute Ventilation (MV) rate-response sensor uses transthoracic impedance measurements to provide rate adaptive pacing based on respiratory rate and trends. When operating as intended, the transthoracic or MV measurement signal is filtered out and not detected on the EGM.

But when an intermittent lead integrity issue causes high impedance conditions, the MV impedance measurement signal may create an undesirable artifact on the corresponding EGM (atrial or ventricular) and be oversensed by the device. SAM enables the device to quickly detect the undesirable artifact and to determine the source of the high impedance. When SAM identifies an event, it creates the episode [1] with impedance measurements and EGM (**Figure 37a**). It remedies the issue by either switching the MV measurement vector (atrial or ventricular) or disabling the MV sensor. In this case, there is no obvious abnormality with the impedance measurements.

2. SAM software changed the MV measurement vector from "A" (atrial ring to can) to "V" (ventricular ring to can) as shown [2] in the before and after parameters (**Figures 37b** and **37c**).

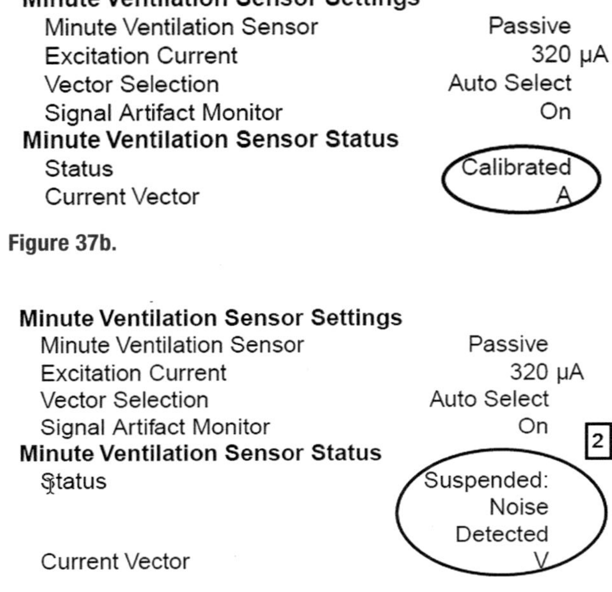

Figure 37b.

Figure 37c.

3. **Figure 37d** is an independent example (from a different patient) of actual oversensed artifact cause by the atrial MV transthoracic impedance signal [3]. Notice that while the artifact has a regular interval (~50 ms), the occurrence and sensing is intermittent. The initial increase in lead impedance is thought to be oxidation of small metal fragments produced by lead and header mismatch (lead and generator are from different manufacturers). The MV signal is normally not seen when the impedance is low and is created by a small, constant current. When impedance is increased and current is constant (Ohm's law, $V = IR$), the resulting applied voltage is higher, producing large signals on the sensing vector that are oversensed.

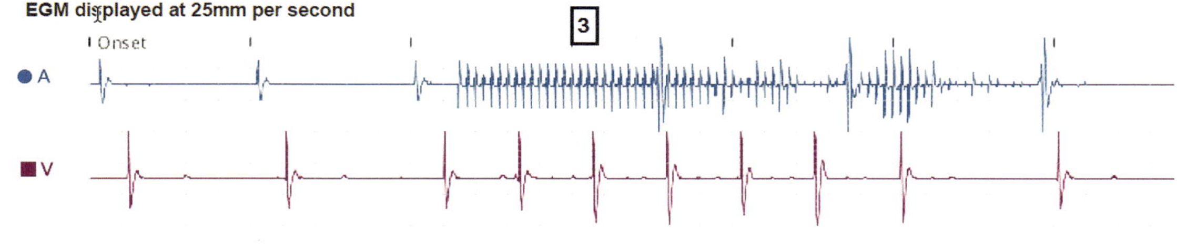

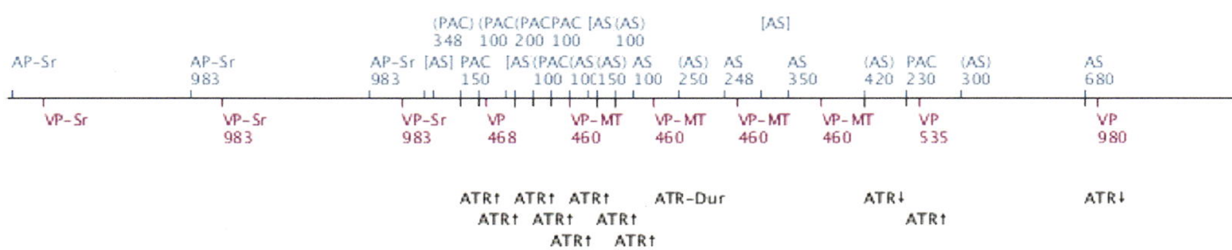

Figure 37d.

4. In this case, SAM actually detected fine atrial flutter as shown in this ATR episode (**Figure 37e**). The atrial flutter interval is regular and at a physiologic (~200 ms) rate [4]. It is appropriately sensed by the ATR and the device is mode switched.

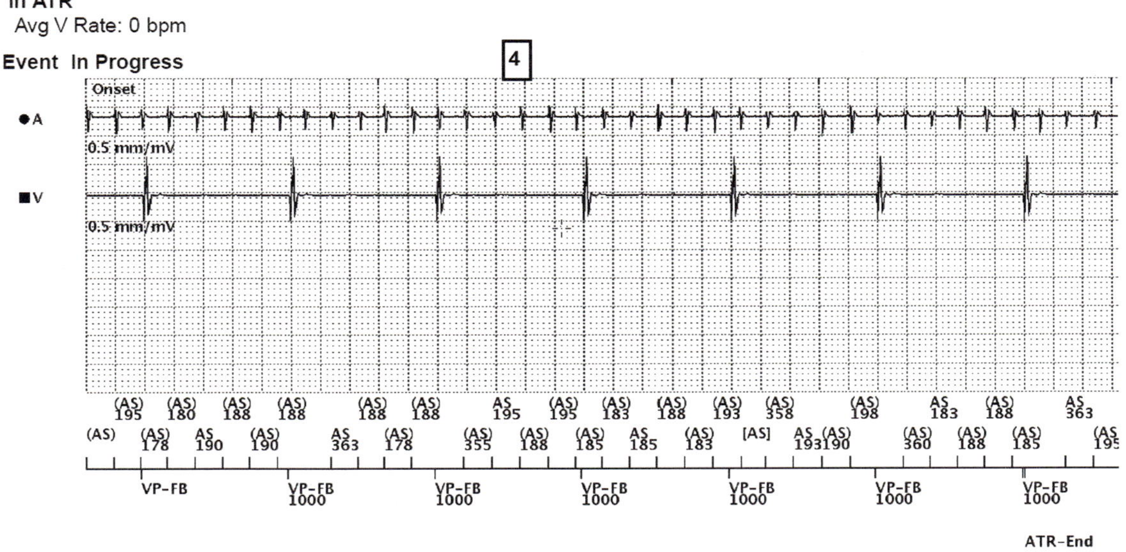

Figure 37e.

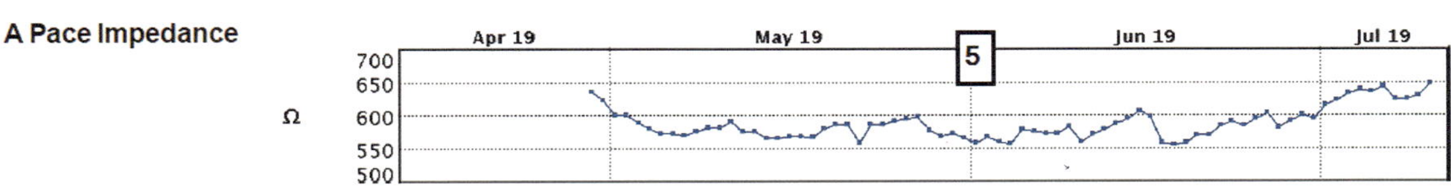

Figure 37f.

5. Another clue is the fact that the impedance measurements at the time of artifact [5] (**Figure 37f**) are all within normal limits. The atrial impedance trend is also stable within normal variations and is missing the telltale abrupt spikes in impedance. This was a false-positive occurrence of transthoracic impedance signal noise by SAM.

CLINICAL RESPONSE

The clinical impact to this patient was minimal. The device unnecessarily changed the MV transthoracic signal vector from the atrial lead to the ventricular lead. The MV sensor will recalibrate using the ventricular lead to measure transthoracic impedance. In the case of both atrial and ventricular lead noise detected by SAM, the MV sensor should be disabled to prevent future oversensing.

38 | Ventricular Noise Reversion

DEVICE: St. Jude Medical* Unify Assura 3357-40 CRT-D

PATIENT: A 79-year-old male received a CRT-D five years earlier for ischemic cardiomyopathy. This patient is also pacemaker-dependent following an atrioventricular node ablation for treatment of chronic atrial fibrillation. He had a non-MRI conditional system, and he underwent a brain MRI for neurological symptoms. How would you interpret the EGM that was collected during the MRI scan in **Figure 38a**? (The programmed parameters are shown in **Figure 38b**.) The EGM and parameters represent the programming and events during the MRI scan.

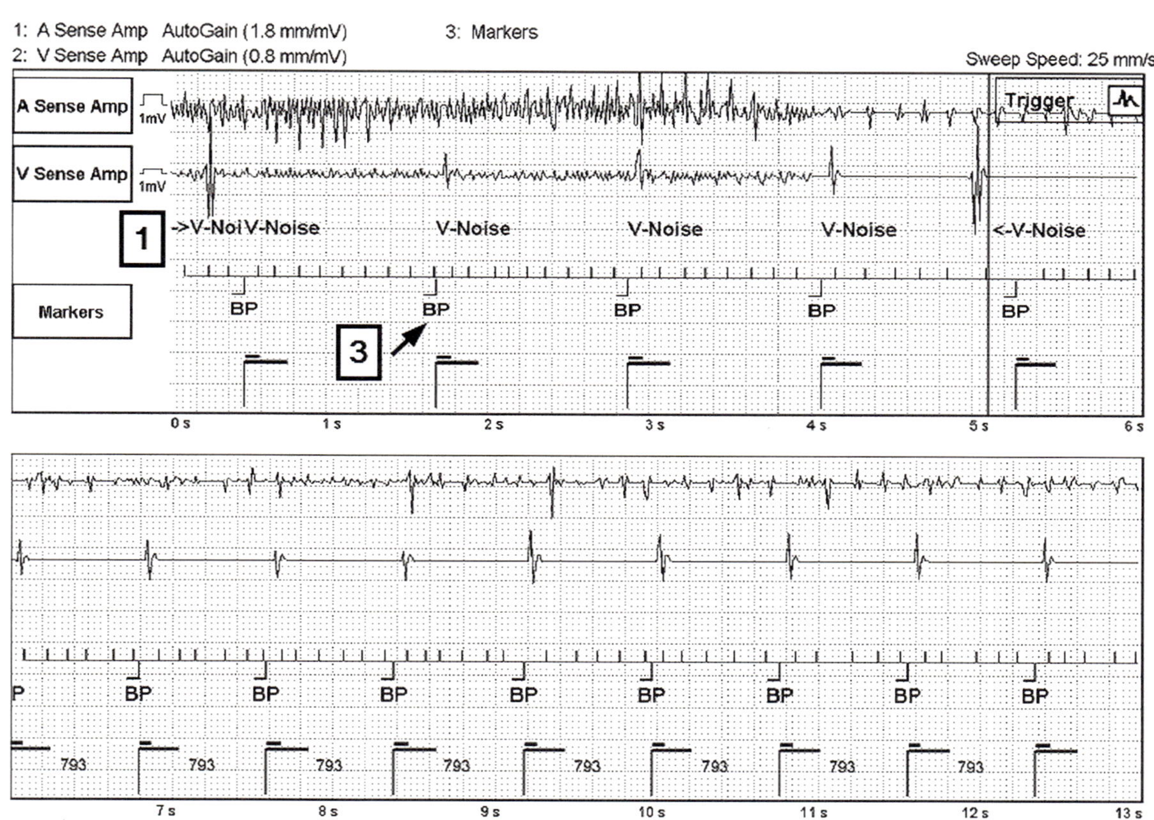

Figure 38a.

---

*St. Jude Medical is now Abbott.

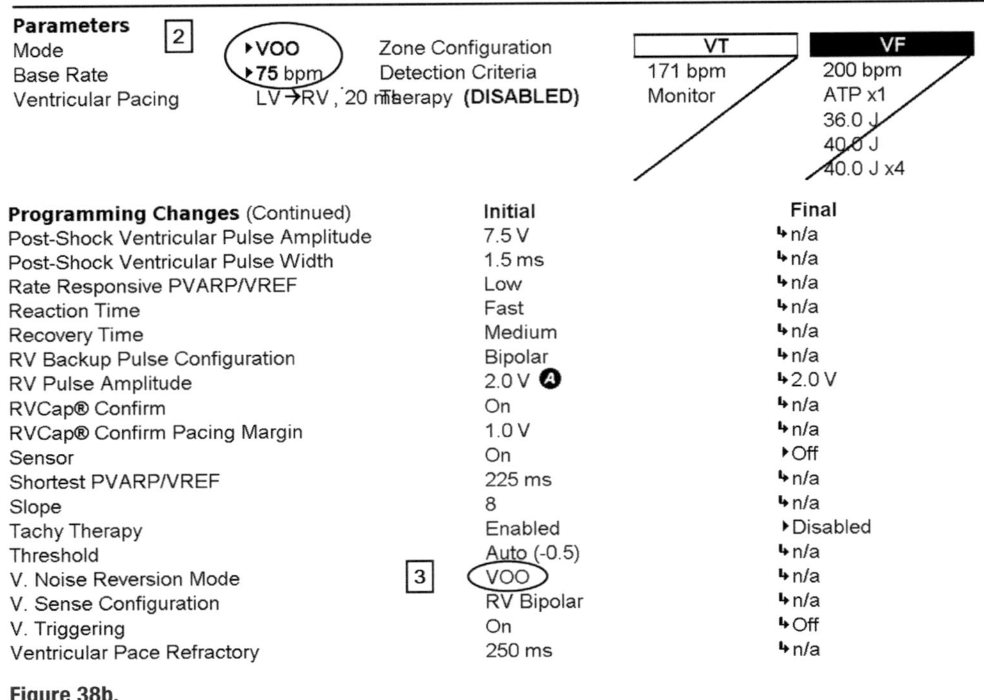

Figure 38b.

ANALYSIS

1. The atrial and ventricular EGMs both show high frequency and regular R waves, and the marker "V-Noise" marks the beginning of the noise reversion mode. The device does not show the ventricular marker channel of these sensed events due to the algorithm detecting "V-noise." In this algorithm, any interval that is sensed on the ventricular channel that exceeds a cycle length of 50 MHz or faster triggers the noise reversion.

2. During the noise reversion, the device performs in a Ventricular (V) Noise Reversion Mode of VOO or OFF. Even though the ICD was programmed to the pacing mode of VOO at 75 bpm [2] for the MRI scan, the V Noise Reversion Mode is still running in the background and detected noise during the MRI scan.

3. When the V Noise Reversion Mode is triggered, and V Noise Reversion mode is set to VOO, the device changes the lower rate limit from the programmed limit of 75 bpm to 50 bpm for the duration of the noise detection. Once V Noise detection has ended, the device reverts to the permanent programmed lower rate limit of 75 bpm. The V Noise Reversion Mode rate cannot be programmed. In the given tracing, the first and the last large signals on RV channel (V sense) are most likely PVCs. In the middle of the tracings, there are R waves following BiV pacing at 50 bpm. There is a delay from the pacing spike to the RV signal on the catheter as LV is paced first (LV–RV delay of 20 ms).

The patient was asymptomatic during the MRI during the change in pacing rate and tolerated the MRI well. The V Noise Reversion Mode parameter needs to be taken into consideration based on the patient's underlying rhythm. If someone is pacemaker-dependent and V. Noise Reversion Mode is set to OFF, and the noise signals are sensed by the device, pacing will be inhibited, which could be detrimental if ventricular asystole ensued.

39 | Ventricular Oversensing with RV Lead Failure

DEVICE: Boston Scientific Inogen EL D141 SC ICD

PATIENT: A 59-year-old female, who has known history of out-of-hospital cardiac arrest, severe multivessel coronary artery disease, and status post single-chamber ICD for secondary prevention was lost to follow-up for a period of time. When communication resumed, the clinic received multiple remote monitor alert transmissions sent for ventricular pacing lead impedance out-of-range (>3000 ohms) as shown in **Figure 39a** and for therapy delivered to convert detected fast rhythm. The EGM recording in **Figure 39b** is typical of several episodes accompanying alert remote transmissions. Shock impedance is also elevated.

Leads	Implant (Jan 15, 2016)	Most Recent In-Office Measurement (Apr 18, 2016)	Most Recent Daily Measurement (Mar 10, 2019)
Ventricular			
Intrinsic Amplitude	17.0 mV	>25.0 mV	>25.0 mV
Pace Impedance	750 Ω	619 Ω	❗ >3000 Ω
Pace Threshold	0.7 V @ 0.5 ms	0.9 V @ 0.4 ms	
Shock			
Shock Impedance	N/R	45 Ω	❗ >200 Ω

Figure 39a.

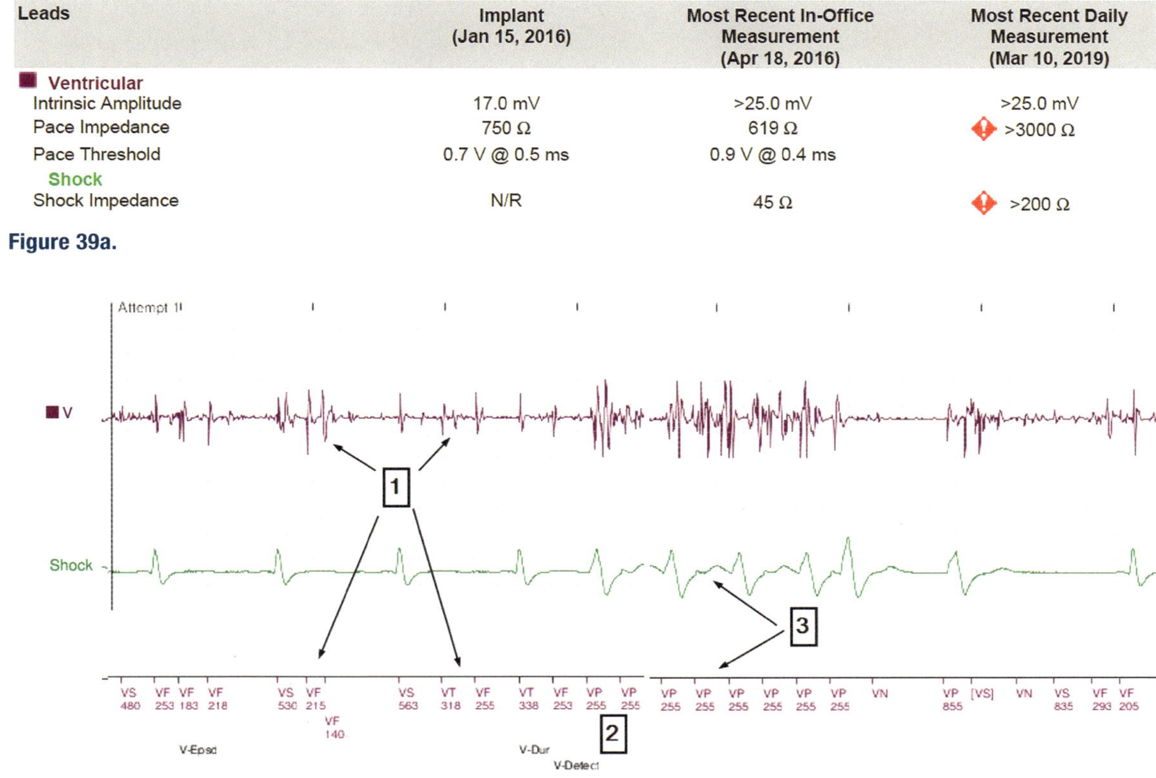

Figure 39b.

ANALYSIS

1. Oversensing of artifact seen on ventricular bipolar channel (RVtip to RVring). The far-field or "shock" EGM channel (RV coil to can) reveals actual ventricular activity without artifact. Intermittent, high-frequency signals with high impedance points to a cable fracture.

2. Ventricular tachycardia detection is met.

3. The device delivers ATP therapy. Failure to 1:1 capture of the ATP is also observed based on the shock EGM. The shock vector also seems to be elevated. This is further evidence of lead failure.

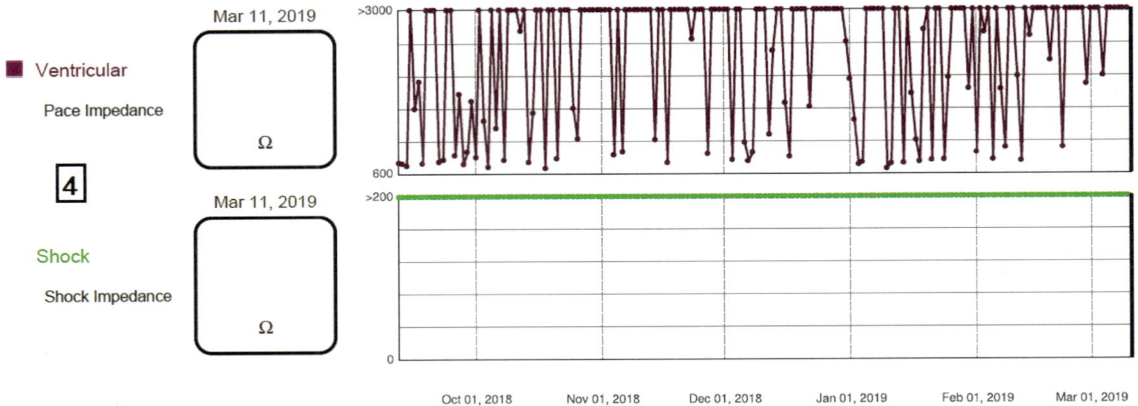

Figure 39c.

4. The RV lead trends also reveal the extent of RV lead failure over an extended period of time.

CLINICAL RESPONSE

The patient received 12 ATP therapies and 0 shocks. After exhaustive attempts at scheduling clinical follow-up, the patient refused care. The patient stated she would seek follow-up at another clinic. Impedance elevation of both the pacing (integrated bipolar vector) and shock components point to conductor cable fracture to the RV coil or a defect at the level of the header where multiple components of the system can be affected.

40 | Atrial Oversensing

DEVICE: Boston Scientific Punctua N051 CRT-D

PATIENT: A 76-year-old congestive heart failure (CHF) patient has a history of paroxysmal atrial fibrillation. The patient had undergone AV node ablation and implantation of a CRT-D device and is pacemaker-dependent. Routine remote follow-up indicated atrial tachycardia events; the EGM tracing from the remote follow-up is shown below in **Figure 40**. What aspects of the EGMs will allow you to determine if this truly represents an atrial tachyarrhythmia?

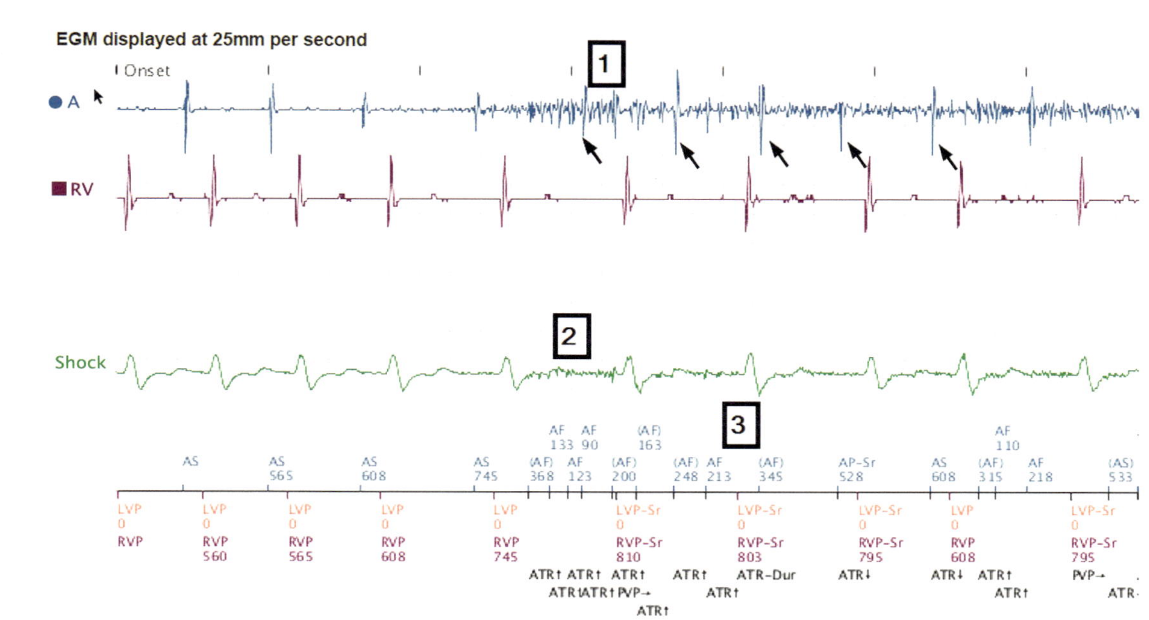

Figure 40.

ANALYSIS

1. High-frequency artifact is shown on the atrial EGM [1]. When the artifact has multiple spikes or up-and-down waves in a very short duration of time, it is referred to as high frequency. It is also sometimes referred to as nonphysiologic. The patterns of the waves do not resemble patterns we would expect from physiologic sources such as heart muscle. On closer inspection, you can observe the more regular, likely intrinsic, sinus EGM pattern through the artifact (indicated by arrows).

2. High-frequency artifact is also seen on the EGM labeled Shock [2]. The shock EGM is a far-field EGM that is created by sensing between RV coil and can. The shock EGM gives you a broader view of any electrical activity. It helps discriminate physiologic and

nonphysiologic sources of electrical activity. In this case, the presence of the high-frequency noise on the shock EGM helps us rule out an atrial lead integrity issue.

3. Oversensing of artifact is noted by the atrial markers. The device is counting some of the artifact spikes in addition to the intrinsic EGM waves. Inappropriate counting toward atrial tachycardia mode switch is indicated by the ATR markers.

CLINICAL RESPONSE

When noise artifact is observed on more than one channel, it may suggest that the source of the noise is outside the device system. If a single lead malfunctions, you would only expect artifact on the one EGM channel associated with the failing lead. As a result of the artifact oversensing discovered on the remote transmission, the patient was brought into the clinic for further follow-up. All in-clinic lead testing was within normal limits. Isometric arm maneuvers reproduced the oversensed artifact. In the absence of any other type of interference, this simple test indicates oversensing of myopotentials as the likely source of interference. Sinus P waves measure 6 mV; atrial fibrillatory waves (actual myopotentials) measured approximately 1.5 mV on atrial EGM. The atrial sensitivity programming was changed from 0.3 mV to 0.7 mV in order to avoid the myopotential sensing, while still appropriately sensing the sinus node and atrial arrhythmia.

41 | Noise Oversensing

DEVICE: St. Jude Medical* Anthem 3210 CRT-P

PATIENT: An 85-year-old female received a dual-chamber CRT-P device 8 years earlier at another institution for sinus node dysfunction and an underlying ischemic cardiomyopathy. The tracing below was obtained on routine remote transmission (**Figure 41a**). Programmed parameters at the time of the remote transmission are shown in **Figure 41b**, and a list of captured episodes is shown in **Figure 41c**. Are true tachyarrhythmias being detected?

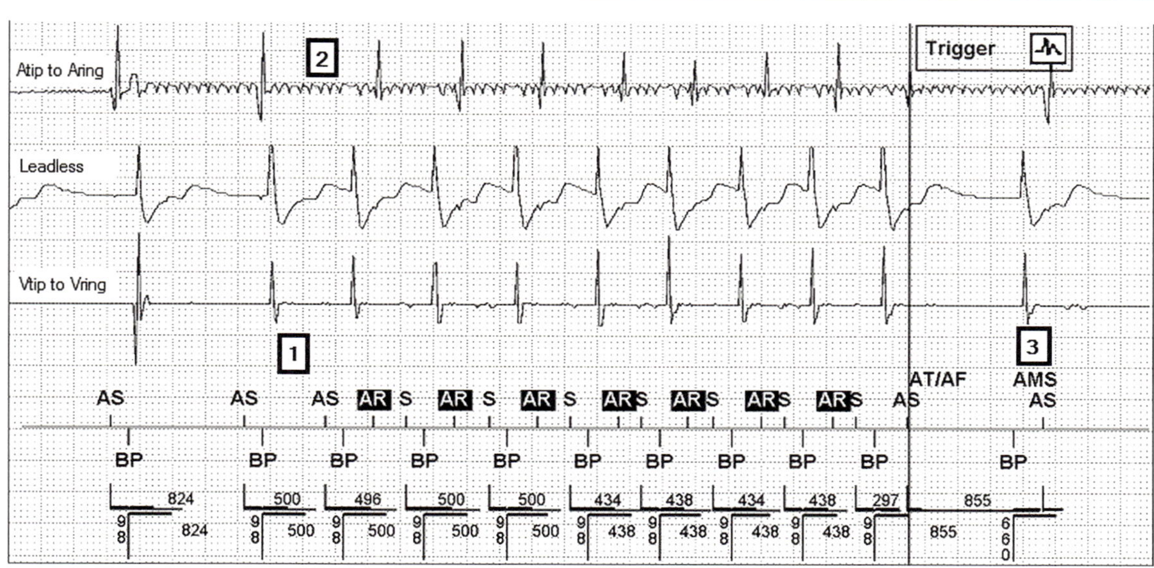

Figure 41a.

Key Parameters

Mode	DDD
Base Rate	50 bpm
Rest Rate	Off
Paced AV Delay	150 ms
Sensed AV Delay	100 ms
Max Track Rate	140 bpm
Max Sensor Rate	140 bpm
Hysteresis Rate	Off
ACap® Confirm	Monitor
RVCap® Confirm	Off
LVCap™ Confirm	On
AF Suppression™	Off
Negative AV Hysteresis/Search	Off
Rate Responsive AV Delay	Off
Rate Responsive PVARP/V Ref	Low
Ventricular Safety Standby	On

Figure 41b.

*St. Jude Medical is now Abbott.

Episodes			
Date / Time	Type	Peak A / V Rate (bpm)	Duration (D:H:M:S)
Jun 13, 2019 7:55 am	AT/AF Detection	244 / 86	0:00:00:10
Jun 12, 2019 3:55 pm	AT/AF Detection	229 / 85	0:00:00:12
Jun 11, 2019 6:55 am	AT/AF Detection	226 / 85	0:00:00:10
Jun 9, 2019 7:55 am	AT/AF Detection	256 / 88	0:00:00:10
Jun 5, 2019 6:55 am	AT/AF Detection	284 / 90	0:00:00:12
Jun 1, 2019 11:55 pm	AT/AF Detection	205 / 81	0:00:00:10
May 29, 2019 6:55 am	AT/AF Detection	244 / 83	0:00:00:12
May 28, 2019 6:55 pm	AT/AF Detection	208 / 82	0:00:00:12
May 28, 2019 5:55 pm	AT/AF Detection	223 / 86	0:00:00:10
May 28, 2019 4:55 pm	AT/AF Detection	256 / 88	0:00:00:10
May 28, 2019 7:55 am	AT/AF Detection	210 / 87	0:00:00:12
May 27, 2019 7:55 am	AT/AF Detection	265 / 87	0:00:00:10
May 24, 2019 7:55 am	AT/AF Detection	233 / 84	0:00:00:10
May 20, 2019 7:55 am	AT/AF Detection	216 / 89	0:00:00:10
May 19, 2019 7:55 am	AT/AF Detection	n/a / n/a	
May 19, 2019 1:55 am	AT/AF Detection	n/a / n/a	
May 19, 2019 12:55 am	AT/AF Detection	n/a / n/a	
May 18, 2019 11:55 pm	AT/AF Detection	n/a / n/a	
May 18, 2019 7:55 am	AT/AF Detection	n/a / n/a	
Apr 27, 2019 6:55 am	AT/AF Detection	240 / 87	0:00:00:10

Figure 41c.

ANALYSIS

1. Markers on the EGM indicate an atrial tachyarrhythmia with frequent events declared as occurring in the atrial refractory period (AR) [1]. The AR events likely represent retrograde P waves that fall into the PVARP. The next sensed A (S) results in tracked BiV pacing. As there is no true atrial contraction prior to BiV pacing, a retrograde A event occurs.

2. The atrial EGM reveals persistent noise on the baseline after the first atrial event [2].

3. As a result of what the device perceives as an atrial tachyarrhythmia, mode switch criteria are met [3].

CLINICAL RESPONSE

Review of all of the available EGMs revealed the same finding, i.e., no true atrial arrhythmia but rather atrial oversensing of noise during a device impedance test. Examining Figure 41c carefully reveals that all of the episodes occurred at 55 minutes after the hour, a clue that something is happening during an automatic internal test of the device.

The manufacturer was contacted; they felt that the device was oversensing a high-frequency "current" signal associated with routine diagnostic impedance measurements. The atrial oversensing resulted in a period of tracking, which was then terminated with the mode switch.

Further investigation revealed that the patient had been seen elsewhere and the atrial sensitivity, which had been at 1.0 mV, was reprogrammed to 0.75 mV.

The patient stated that she had been asymptomatic, i.e., she was not aware of these episodes. She was brought into the device clinic where the atrial sensitivity was reprogrammed to 1.0 mV, which eliminated further noise oversensing.

42 | Electromagnetic Interference in ICD

DEVICE: Medtronic Evera XT DR DDBB1D1 DC ICD

PATIENT: A 59-year-old patient with a history of Ebstein's anomaly and moderately severe right ventricular dysfunction received an ICD for recurrent ventricular tachycardia. The patient sent a remote transmission because his device was beeping and he had received a shock while in a swimming pool. EGMs from the remote transmission are shown in **Figures 42a** and **42b**. Was the shock real and was it appropriate?

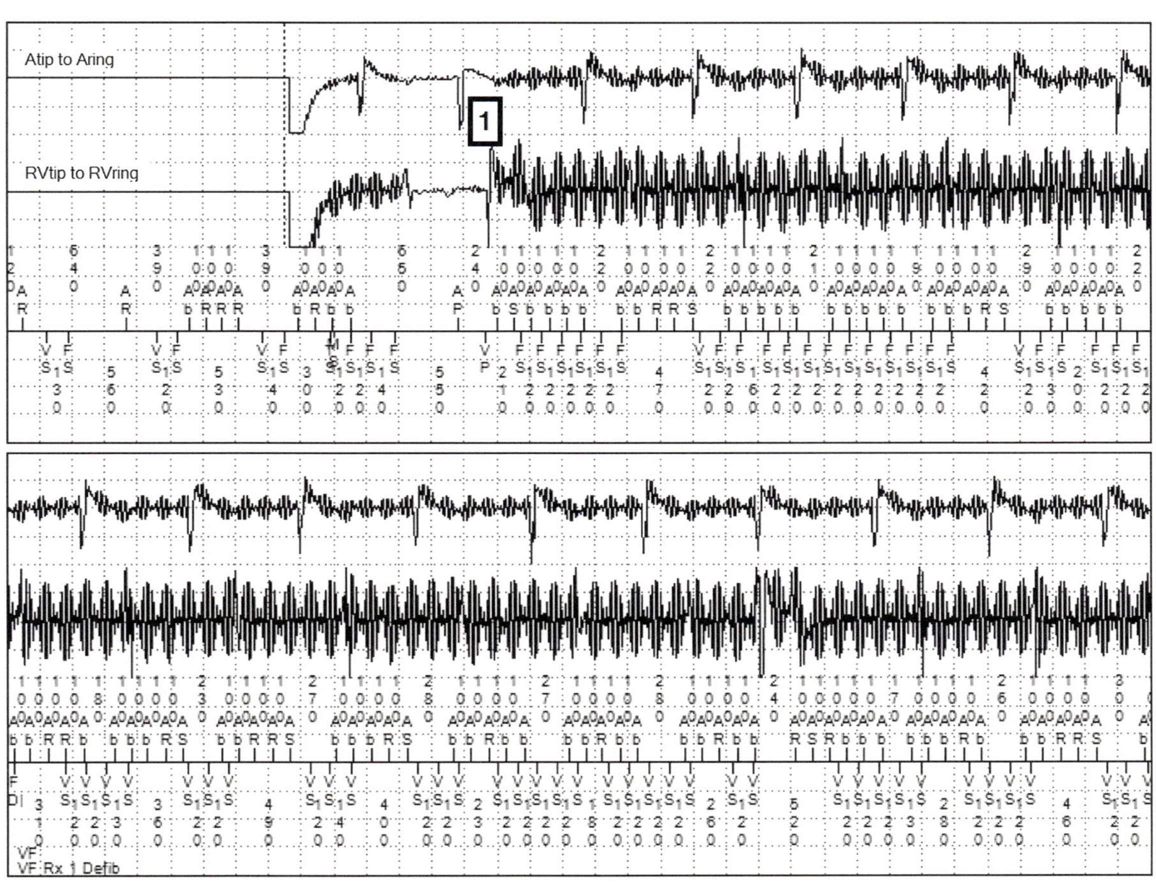

Figure 42a.

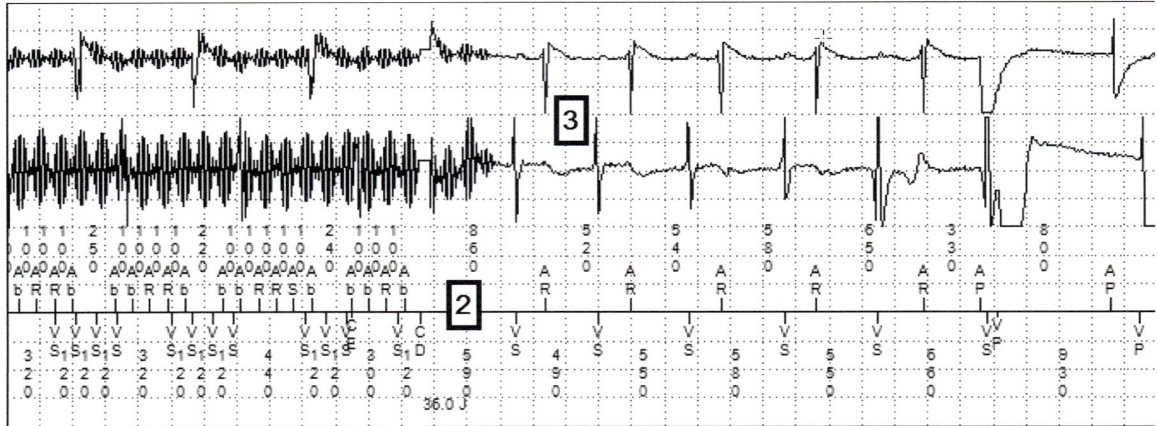

Figure 42b.

ANALYSIS

1. The EGM in Figure 42a demonstrates high-frequency, continuous signals on both atrial and ventricular channels. The signals most likely represent electromagnetic interference (EMI) on both the atrial channel and ventricular channels. This phenomenon occurs when some aspect of the electrical system supporting the swimming pool is not grounded (light source, pump, or pool-cleaning robots). Most commonly, it is from an underwater light that is not appropriately grounded. Stray voltage circulating through the water created noise on both leads due to the fact the lights within the pool was not grounded. For the signals to be appropriately displayed on the tracings they should be sampled at twice the frequency of interested signals. In the United States, the frequency of AC current is 60 Hz, and when 128 Hz sampling is used for telemetry, an 8 Hz beat frequency (128–120 Hz) is noted on the signals. The beat frequency is appreciated well on the RV channel with intervals of 120 ms.

2. In Figure 42b, the device interprets the EMI as an actual ventricular arrhythmia and as a result charges and delivers an inappropriate 36-J shock. The patient was exiting the pool when this happened.

3. The majority of waveforms in Figure 42b coincides with the patient exiting the pool and away from the EMI source of the stray current.

CLINICAL RESPONSE

The patient went to his local emergency department (ED) because of the continued beeping from the device. The beeping was appropriate because the device was programmed to alert the patient when the device delivered a shock. In the ED, the device was interrogated, and the alert tone was turned off. The patient was instructed not to swim in that pool until the electrical system was appropriately grounded.

43 | RV Lead Failure

DEVICE: St. Jude Medical* Fortify Assura VR 1357-40C SC ICD

PATIENT: A 15-year-old patient required an epicardial ICD system 5 years earlier for primary prevention after diagnosis of long QT syndrome.

The lead impedance trend over the preceding year (**Figure 43a**) and EGM (**Figure 43b**) shown below are from a Merlin remote transmission after the patient received a vibratory alert. A sudden increase in impedance value that is sustained is highly suspect for complete lead fracture.

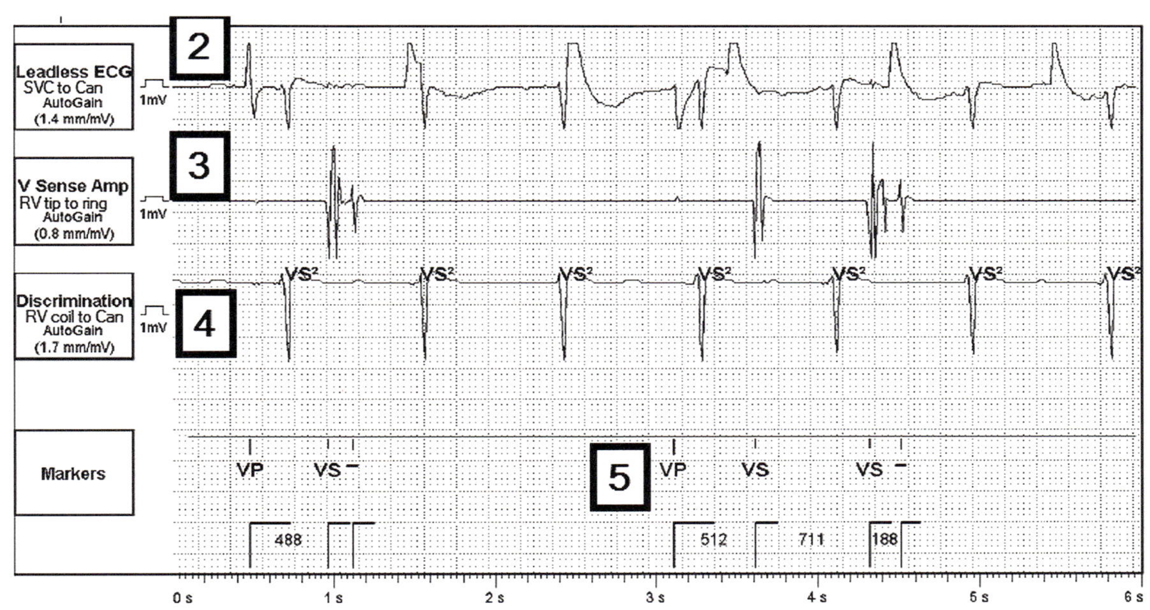

Figure 43a.

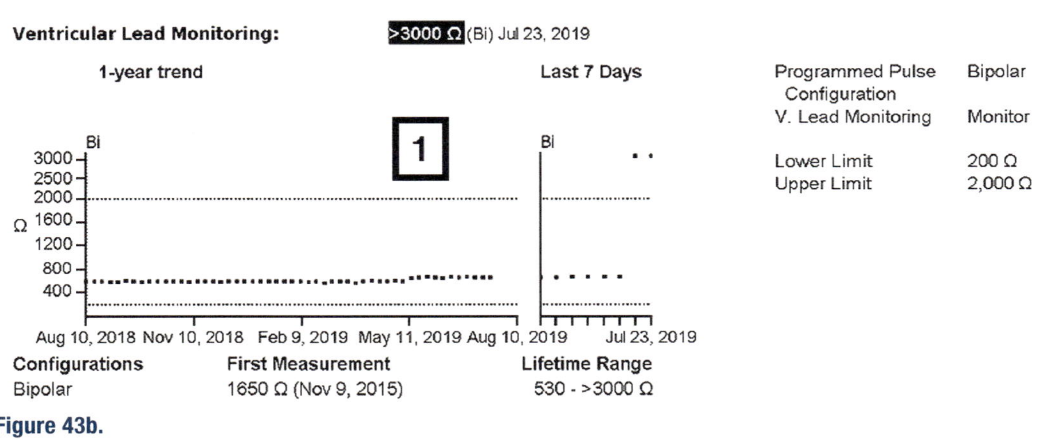

Figure 43b.

*St. Jude Medical is now Abbott.

ANALYSIS

1. The most recent RV pace impedance at time of remote transmission was >3000 ohms. When looking at the last year trends, impedance appears to have been stable in the 500 to 600 ohms range until an abrupt increase was seen on the last two daily measurements. This acute, abrupt increase in lead impedance is suspicious for lead fracture.

2. The leadless EGM is configured SVC to can, but this device does not have a lead plugged into the SVC coil port (SVC port is plugged with a pin). As a result, the leadless EGM is inaccurate [2]. The leadless EGM is customizable through programming to avoid the SVC port, but in this case, the nominal settings were not changed.

3. The RV EGM is tip to ring [3] and is predominantly isoelectric with occasional high frequency alternating R waves. Comparing the near-field RV EGM to the discrimination EGM, there is a discrepancy, as the discrimination EMG appears to show regular R waves at approximately 75 bpm whereas the near-field EGM has cycle intervals that are variable and short enough to start a bin toward a tachycardia therapy zone.

4. Discrimination EGM [4] senses RV coil to can so that the device can compare the near-field EGM to the discrimination EGM. This allows for another discriminator that is used when a tachyarrhythmia is detected to prevent inappropriate shocks from oversensing. The VS^2 marker on the discrimination channel represents a ventricular sensed event via RV coil to can.

5. Due to the failure of the device to sense both patient's intrinsic heart rhythm and any noise, the lower rate limit was reached at 30 bpm and a VP was delivered. The corresponding VP marker when compared to the discriminator channel reveals that the paced beat did not capture as there is no immediate paced R wave following the VP marker. It is more common to see noise after pacing or after shock therapy delivery

CLINICAL RESPONSE

The evidence of undersensing, oversensing, loss of capture from a ventricular pace, as well as an abrupt increase in pace impedance are all signs of a lead fracture. The patient was contacted and instructed to be seen urgently for device interrogation and deactivating the ICD functions as well as pacing functions due to the lead fracture and inappropriate functioning. The need to have the patient seen urgently to deactivate the ICD and pacing function would be to prevent inappropriate shock(s). The patient eventually underwent complete replacement of epicardial pacing and defibrillation coil.

44 | RV Lead Fracture

DEVICE: Medtronic Evera XT DR DDBB1D1 DC ICD

PATIENT: A 57-year-old patient has a dual-chamber ICD implanted four years earlier for non-ischemic cardiomyopathy and significantly impaired LV function. The patient initiated a manual remote transmission after hearing an audible alert tone from their ICD. Previous interrogations had revealed stable device and lead measurements. The EGM from the patient-initiated transmission is shown below in **Figure 44a** and impedance measurements in **Figure 44b**.

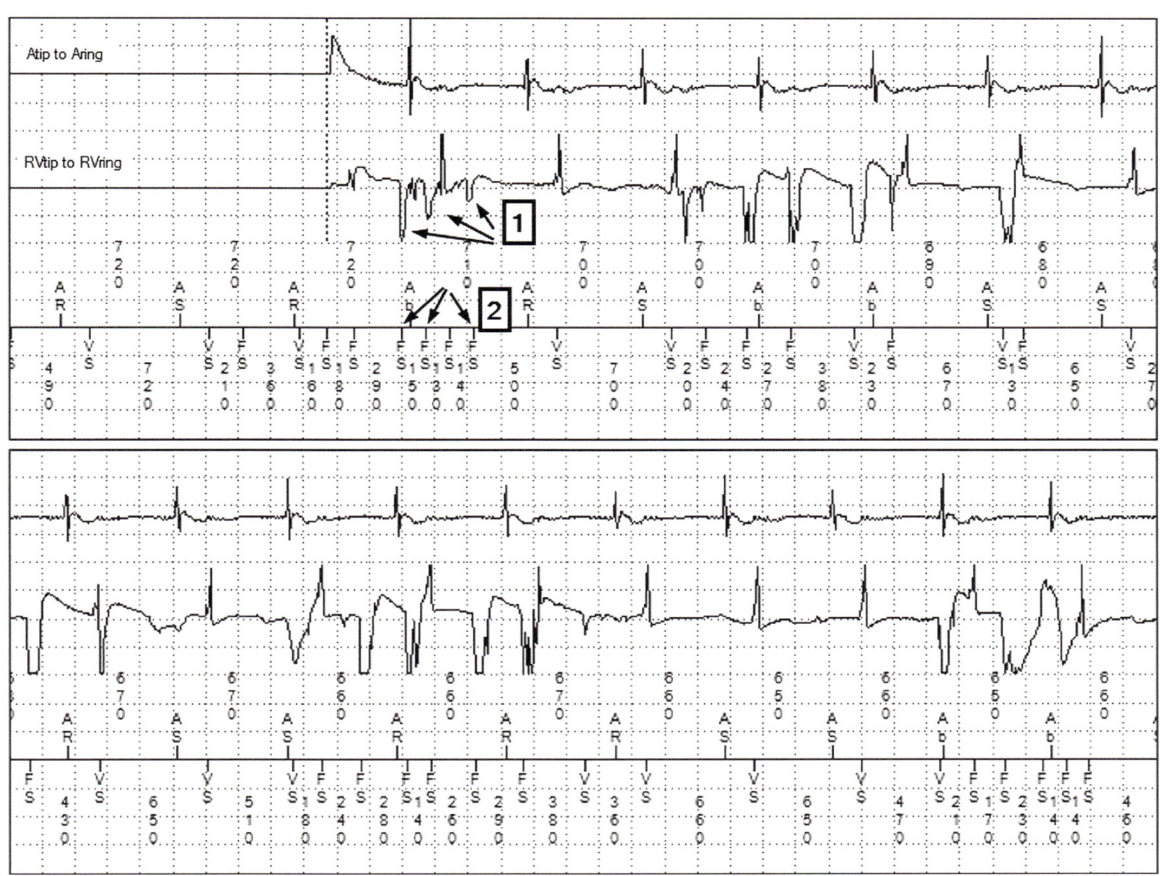

Figure 44a.

Event	Threshold
*RV Bipolar lead impedance >3000 ohms.	3000 ohms
*RVtip to RVcoil lead impedance >3000 ohms.	3000 ohms

Figure 44b.

ANALYSIS

1. When looking at the RV near-field EGM, there are R waves that are erratic, irregular, and inconsistent. There are also R-to-R intervals measured as short as 130 ms or 460 bpm, which would be considered nonphysiologic. Because the erratic and inconsistent R waves are only seen on the RV channel, this eliminates the likelihood of EMI, as it would likely be seen on all leads. Lead noise due to fracture leads to intermittent, high-frequency, nonphysiological signals with occasional amplifier saturation.

2. The nonphysiologic R waves or artifact is being sensed by the device and are counted towards tachycardia detection.

3. CareLink alerts displayed from the remote transmission are in Figure 44b. The RV bipolar (RVtip to RVring) and integrated bipolar (RVtip to RVcoil) impedance values both measured >3000 ohms. Impedance values previously were stable around 600 ohms bipolar and 550 ohms integrated bipolar. The device's audible alert was triggered due to these impedance values during an automated device function test. The RV defibrillation impedance remained stable around 90 ohms. Taking these device measurements and this EGM into consideration, these abnormalities are suspect for a lead fracture, more specifically the conductor cable corresponding to the RV tip.

CLINICAL RESPONSE

The patient was contacted and concerns regarding the transmission results were shared. The patient was instructed to present to the local ED, where the device could be interrogated and ICD therapies programmed OFF until RV lead revision could be completed to prevent inappropriate shocks related to RV lead failure.

45 | Atrial Oversensing with Inappropriate Mode Switch and Arrhythmia Induction

DEVICE: Medtronic Advisa DR MRI A2DR01 DC PM

PATIENT: The patient is a 29-year-old male who was implanted with pacemaker for atrial flutter and is also post AV node ablation. Consider the AT/AF episode in **Figure 45a** reported in routine remote follow-up. The patient was asymptomatic. Atrial ATP therapies are programmed as shown in **Figure 45b**.

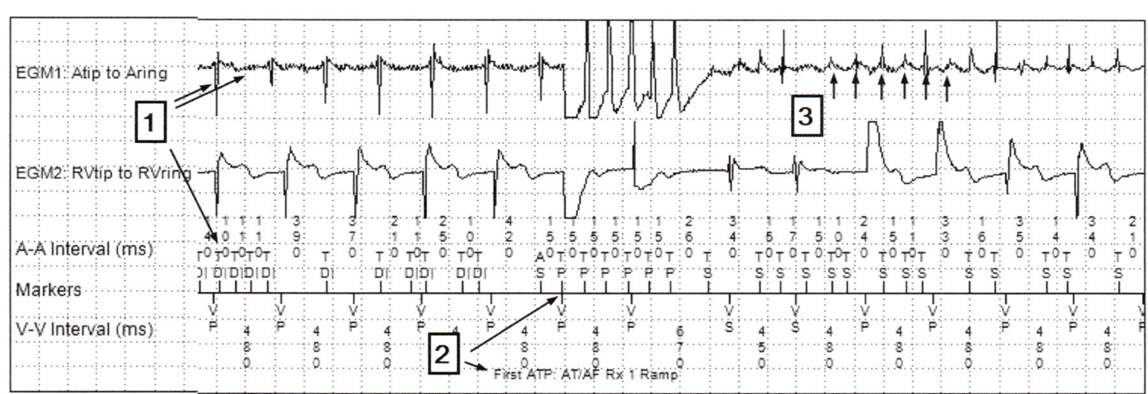

Figure 45a.

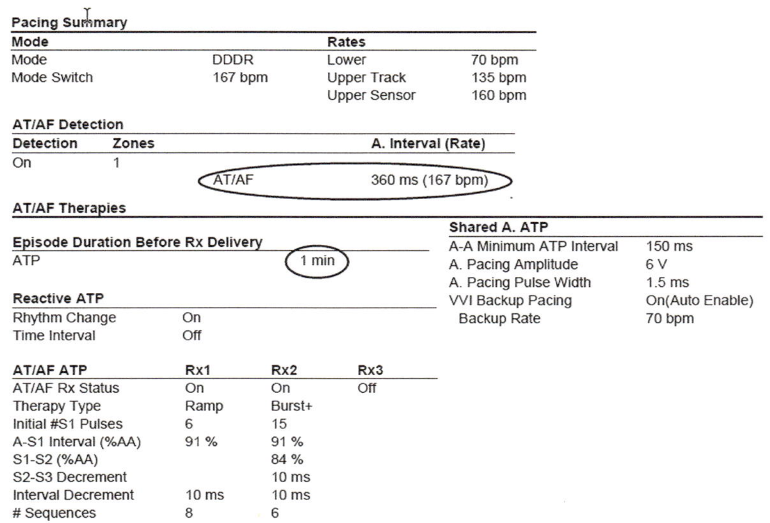

Figure 45b.

1. When atrial therapies are programmed on, the atrial TD channel marker refers to AT/AF detected events. In this case, the device channel markers do not correlate with the atrial EGM [1]. In addition to atrial events (150 bpm) there is oversensing of high-frequency artifact also evident on the atrial EGM.

2. As a result of what the device believes to be an atrial tachyarrhythmia, there is inappropriate delivery of atrial ATP therapy. The oversensed events are counted toward detection and eventualy meet the 167 bpm, with duration of 1 minute required for atrial therapy (Figure 45b). The first ramp ATP therapy is given by the device [2]. Note the ATP interval is fixed at 150 ms despite being programed to RAMP pacing. This is because the atrial oversensing interval is so short, ATP reaches the minimal pacing interval of 150 ms (Figure 45b).

3. Following the atrial ATP therapy there is a change in the atrial EGM. The intrinsic atrial rate changes from 150 bpm to an atrial flutter at greater than 300 bpm. It is likely that the previous inappropriate delivery of atrial ATP during normal sinus rhythm was proarrhythmic.

CLINICAL RESPONSE

Atrial ATP was a successful therapy for this patient. In this situation, the atrial arrhythmia therapy algorithm was counterproductive and proarrhythmic, inducing an atrial episode. The patient was brought into the clinic for full testing of the atrial lead. No obvious abnormalities were found. For a period of time, the atrial lead was observed. There continued to be intermittent episodes of atrial oversensing with inappropriate therapy despite adjustment of atrial sensitivity. The atrial lead was extracted and replaced, with subsequent normal device function.

46 | Short-Long-Short-Induced Ventricular Tachycardia

DEVICE: Boston Scientific Incepta DR E163 DC ICD

PATIENT: A 69-year-old patient with a history of out-of-hospital arrest status post aortic valve replacement, left bundle branch block with intermittent 2:1 AV conduction, and dilated cardiomyopathy received a dual-chamber ICD. The patient had a recent ventricular tachycardia event and received a 41-J shock. The patient was asleep at the time and suddenly awoke with pain and tenderness at the ICD site. Could this event potentially have been prevented?

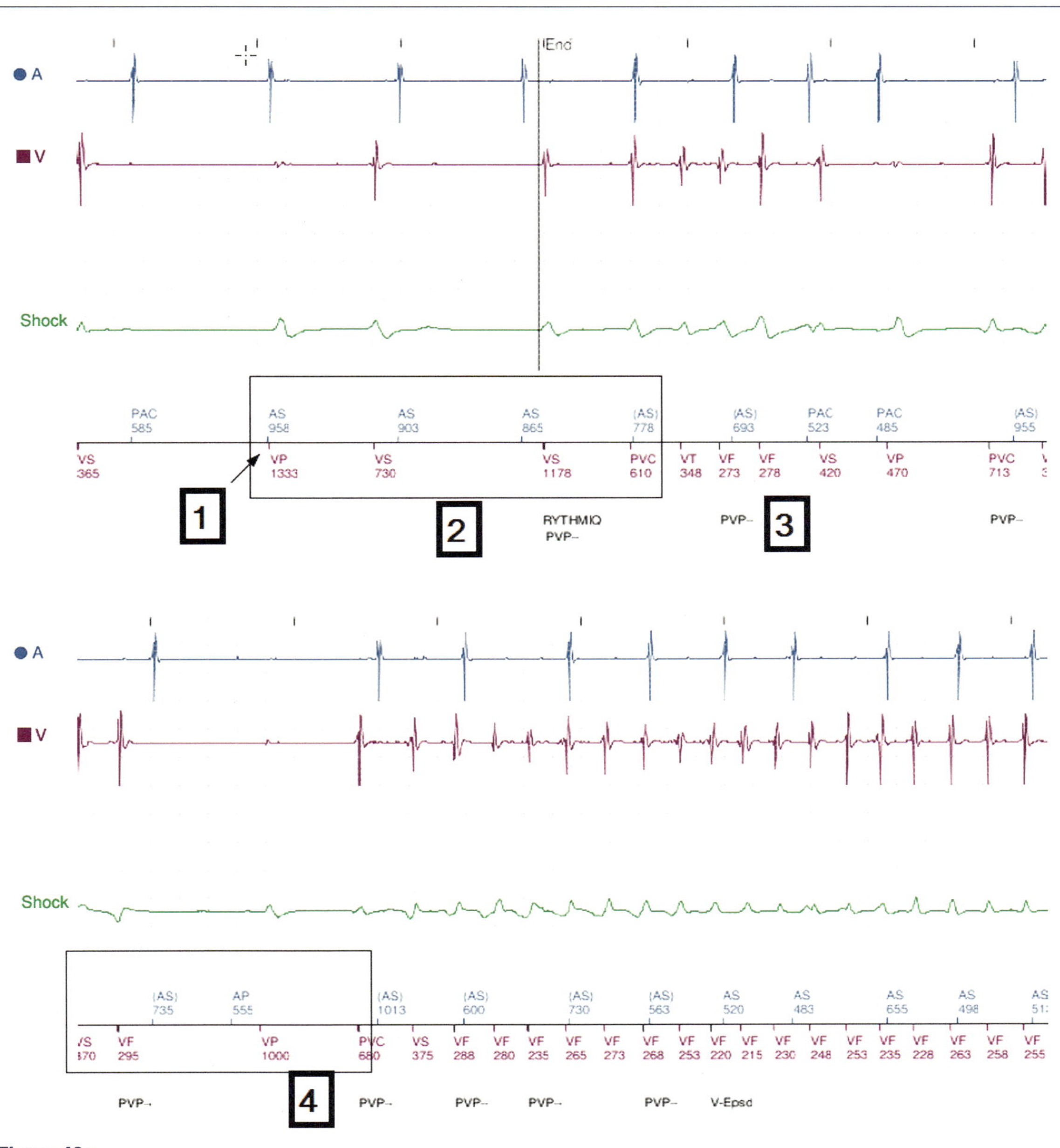

Figure 46a.

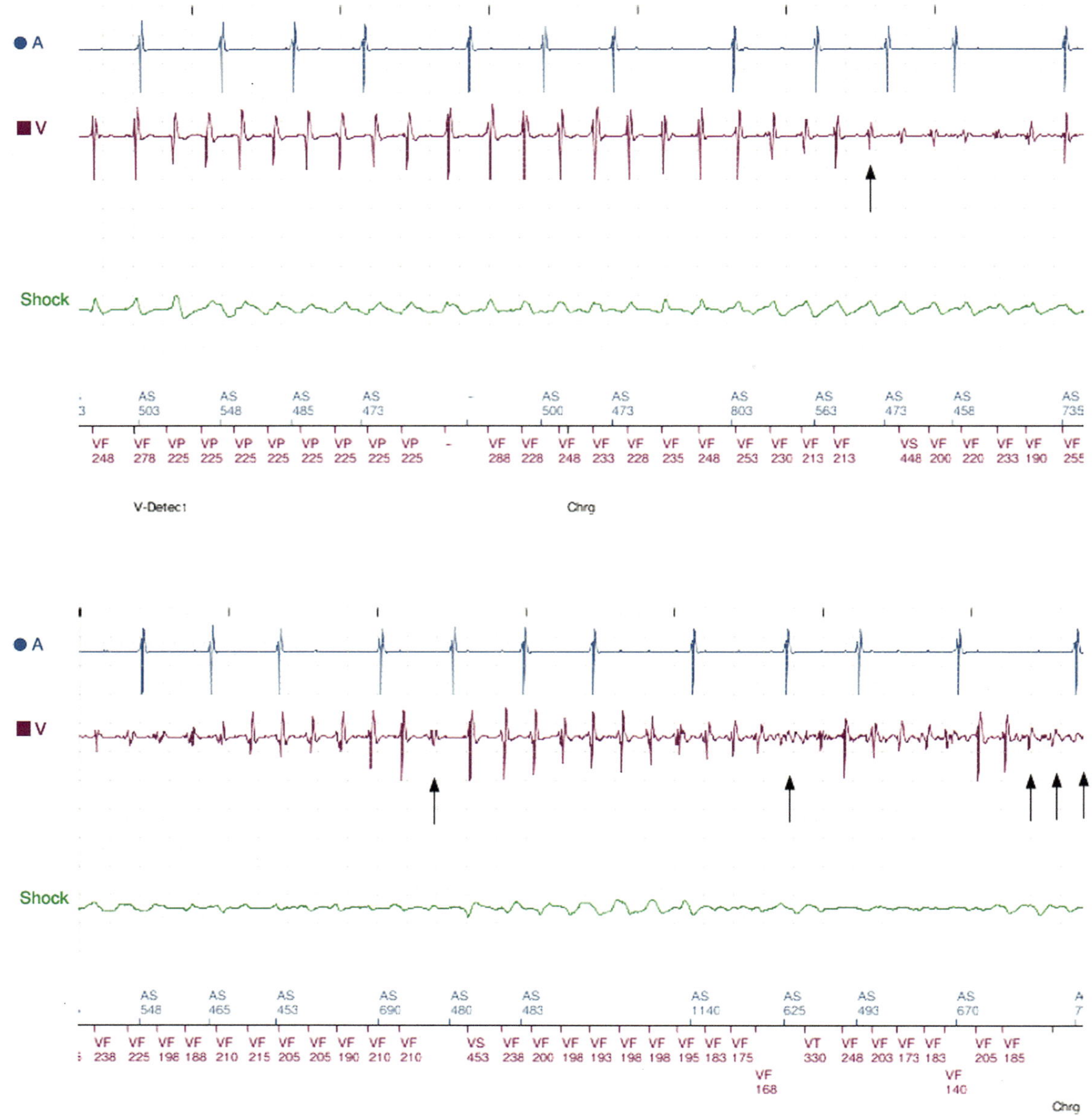

Figure 46b.

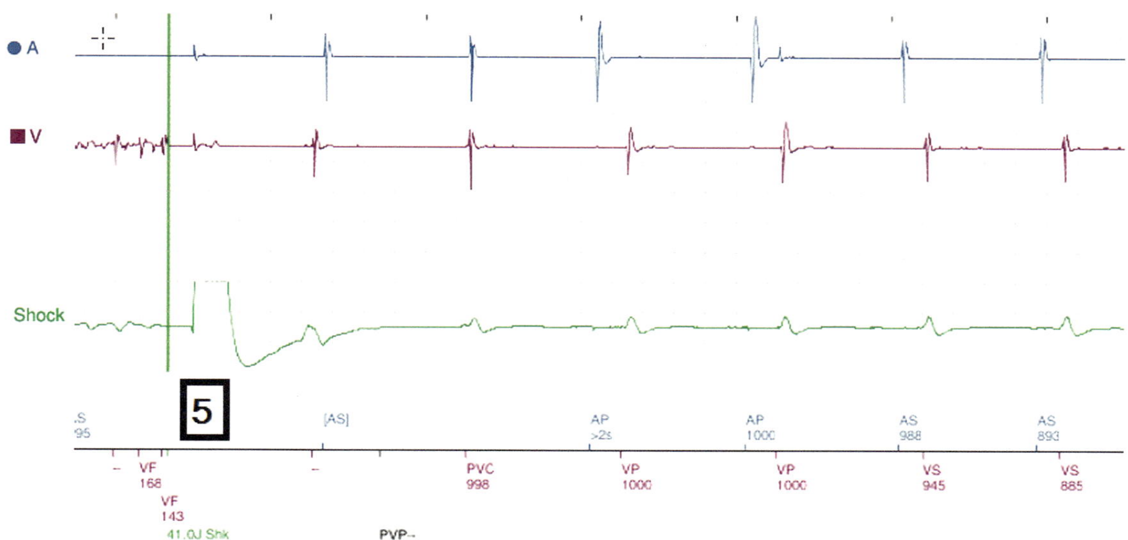

Figure 46c.

Settings

Ventricular Tachy

VF	200 bpm	ATP	41 J, 41 J, 41 Jx6
VT	170 bpm	Monitor Only	

Atrial Tachy

ATR Mode Switch	170 bpm	DDIR	

Pacing Output
- Atrial — 1.5 V @ 0.4 ms
- Ventricular — 2.0 V @ 0.6 ms

Brady

Mode	DDD	
RYTHMIQ™	AAI With VVI Backup	
Lower Rate Limit	60 ppm	
Maximum Tracking Rate	130 ppm	
Maximum Sensor Rate	130 ppm	
Paced AV Delay	80 - 200 ms	
Sensed AV Delay	70 - 170 ms	
A-Refractory (PVARP)	240 - 280 ms	
V-Refractory (VRP)	230 - 250 ms	

Sensitivity
- Atrial — AGC 0.25 mV
- Ventricular — AGC 0.6 mV

Leads Configuration (Pace/Sense)
- Atrial — Bipolar
- Ventricular — Bipolar

Sensor
- Accelerometer — ATR Only

Ventricular Tachy

VF 200 bpm (300 ms)

Detection/Redetection

		Therapy	
Initial Duration	2.5 s	QUICK CONVERT™ ATP	On
Redetection Duration	1.0 s	Shock 1	41 J
Post-shock Duration	1.0 s	Shock 2	41 J
		Additional 41 J Shocks	6

VT 170 bpm (353 ms)

Detection/Redetection

Initial Duration	9.0 s	ATP1	Off
Redetection Duration	1.0 s	Number of Bursts	Off
Post-shock Duration	1.0 s	ATP2	Off
		Number of Bursts	Off

Shocks

Shock 1	Off J
Shock 2	Off J
Shock 3 -6	Off J

Ventricular Tachy Therapy Setup

ATP

		Shock (All Shocks)	
Ventricular ATP Amplitude	7.5 V	Waveform	Biphasic
Ventricular ATP Pulse Width	2.0 ms	Committed Shock	Off

Magnet and Beeper

Magnet Response	Inhibit Therapy	Lead Polarity	Initial
Beep During Capacitor Charge	Off	Shock Lead Vector	RV Coil to Can

Figure 46d.

ANALYSIS

1. In **Figure 46a**, the device paces the ventricle at a rate of 45 bpm due to Boston Scientific's Rythmiq™ algorithm. The Rythmiq works by running two simultaneous modes: AAI, which is at the lower programmed rate, and VVI, which is equivalent to 15 bpm less than the lower rate, which in this case is equal to 45 bpm (60 – 15 = 45 bpm). The Rythmiq

algorithm is designed to minimize ventricular pacing. The morphology of displayed VS and VP events in Boston Scientific devices is quite different due to differential signal processing.

2. Figure 46a illustrates a short-long-short (S-L-S) sequence of ventricular events that trigger nonsustained ventricular tachycardia (NSVT). The S-L-S sequences can amplify beat to beat repolarization changes leading to polymorphic ventricular tachycardia. Algorithms that promote intrinsic conduction can occasionally lead to pauses (S-L-S sequences) that can result in polymorphic VT in certain individuals.

3. In Figure 46a, NSVT was triggered by the S-L-S sequences and self-terminates. The device also ended the Rythmiq algorithm switching to DDDR due to the loss of AV synchrony.

4. In Figure 46a, the EGM illustrates another S-L-S sequence, which this time leads into a polymorphic VT. Then in **Figure 46b**, the EGM demonstrates polymorphic VT, which is detected resulting in the device delivering ATP, which is unsuccessful. The ICD then begins to charge. The rhythm deteriorates to ventricular fibrillation (VF) with some undersensed beats.

5. **Figure 46c** illustrates the device delivering a 41-J shock which terminates the VF with a type I break (clean), restoring sinus rhythm.

6. **Figure 46d** shows the device settings at the time.

CLINICAL RESPONSE

The patient went to her local ED since she did not feel well upon awakening. The patient received electrolyte and fluid replacement and was discharged the following day. The patient was then brought into the clinic, where the device nurse, under the direction of the physician, turned off Rythmiq, lengthened the sensed AV delay to 240 ms, and lengthened the paced AV delay to 260 ms. Since these changes were made, the patient has not had any recurrent episodes.

47 | Managed Ventricular Pacing Mode and Ventricular Arrhythmias

DEVICE: Medtronic Evera XT DR DDBB1D4 DC ICD

PATIENT: A 69-year-old female was admitted to the ED following two ICD shocks. On admission, ECG demonstrated sinus rhythm with one-to-one AV conduction. The QTC was markedly prolonged at around 600 ms. She was found to have hypokalemia with serum potassium of 3.3 mmol/L. Programmed settings are shown in **Figure 47a**. EGMs for an episode are shown below in **Figures 47b** and **47c**. After reviewing the episodes consider whether the AAI ↔ DDD mode contributed to the event.

Pacing Summary

Mode		Rates		AV Intervals	
Mode	AAIR<=>DDDR	Lower	60 bpm	Paced AV	180 ms
Mode Switch	171 bpm	Upper Track	140 bpm	Sensed AV	150 ms
		Upper Sensor	140 bpm		

Refractory/Blanking

PVARP	Auto
Minimum PVARP	250 ms
PVAB Interval	150 ms
PVAB Method	Partial+
A. Blank Post AP	200 ms
A. Blank Post AS	100 ms
V. Blank Post VP	200 ms
V. Blank Post VS	120 ms

VT/VF Detection

		V. Interval (Rate)	Initial	Redetect
VF	On	300 ms (200 bpm)	18/24	12/16
FVT	OFF			
VT	OFF	360 ms (167 bpm)	16	12
Monitor	Monitor	370 ms (162 bpm)	32	

Figure 47a.

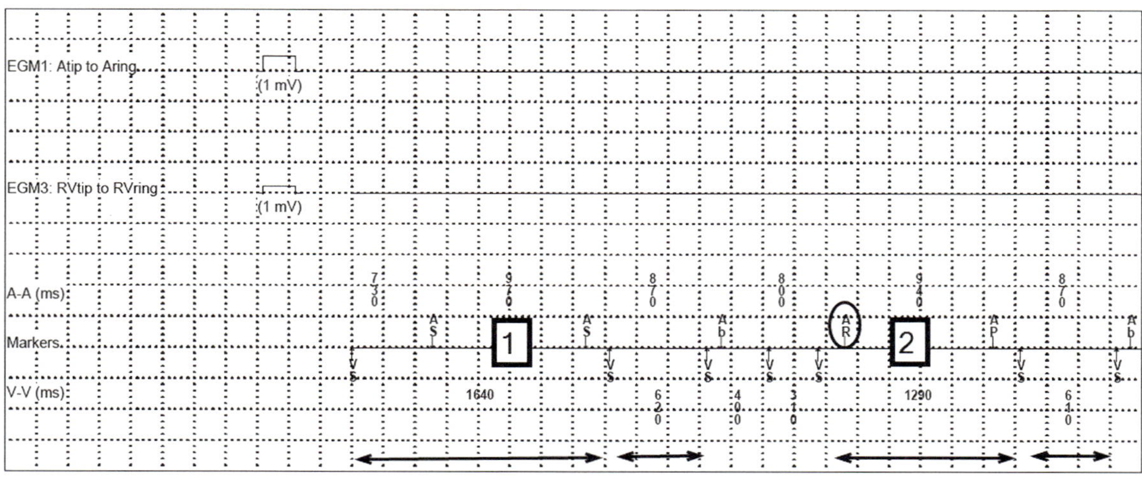

Figure 47b.

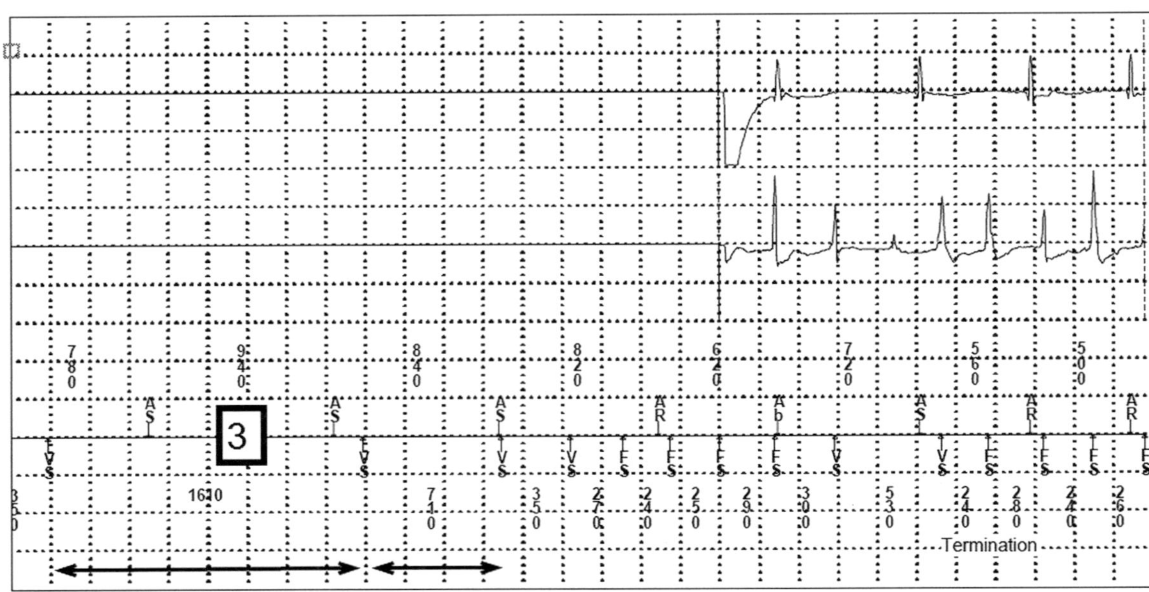

Figure 47c.

ANALYSIS

1. Programmed settings in Figure 47a show the mode AAI ↔ DDD. Medtronic has termed this mode Managed Ventricular Pacing (MVP). It is a V-pacing avoidance algorithm that works in the following way: The device functions in AAI or AAIR mode until it detects that two of the last four A-A intervals do not contain a V-sensed event occurring between the atrial events. When this criterion is met, it switches to either DDD or DDDR mode with the potential to return to AAI or AAIR mode when AV conduction has resumed, for which it periodically checks. The second blocked atrial event (not an "AR" event) triggers ventricular pacing at short AV delay and is not seen in the above tracings.

2. In Figure 47b, the first A-A interval [1] shows no ventricular sensed event occurring between the two atrial events. A second A-A interval without a V-sensed event [2] occurs within the required four A-A intervals, however, this does not trigger the switch to DDD mode because one of the two atrial events fell into refractory (see circled AR). In Figure 47c, another A-A interval without a sensed ventricular event occurs. Once again, this does not trigger a switch to DDD because of the AR event previously mentioned. In this case, the device continues to function in AAI mode.

3. In both figures, the arrows indicate where the loss of AV conduction has led to V-V cycle lengths that alternate between short and long, a known precursor to ventricular arrhythmias, particularly in patients with a long QT interval.

Marked variation in R-R intervals can lead to amplification of the repolarization period. These changes are more pronounced when someone has predisposing factors that prolong repolarization. In this patient, electrolytes were replenished and the device programmed to DDD mode with long AV delays to minimize ventricular pacing.

48 | Ventricular Pacing in the Vulnerable Period Due to Blanking and Associated Arrhythmia

DEVICE: Boston Scientific Energen DR E143 DC ICD

PATIENT: A 63-year-old male was implanted with a dual-chamber ICD following a ventricular fibrillation arrest and coronary artery bypass graft (CABG) surgery. The patient experienced multiple recent episodes of ventricular tachycardia, the majority of which were initiated by PVCs. In the EGMs from the episode shown below in **Figures 48a**, **48b**, **48c**, and **48d**, the precipitating event is atrial pacing followed by ventricular pacing in the vulnerable period after the PVC. Settings are shown in **Figure 48e**. The EGMs in **Figure 48f** is an example of what was seen frequently at the hospital bedside, leading to the programming changes evidenced in **Figure 48g**.

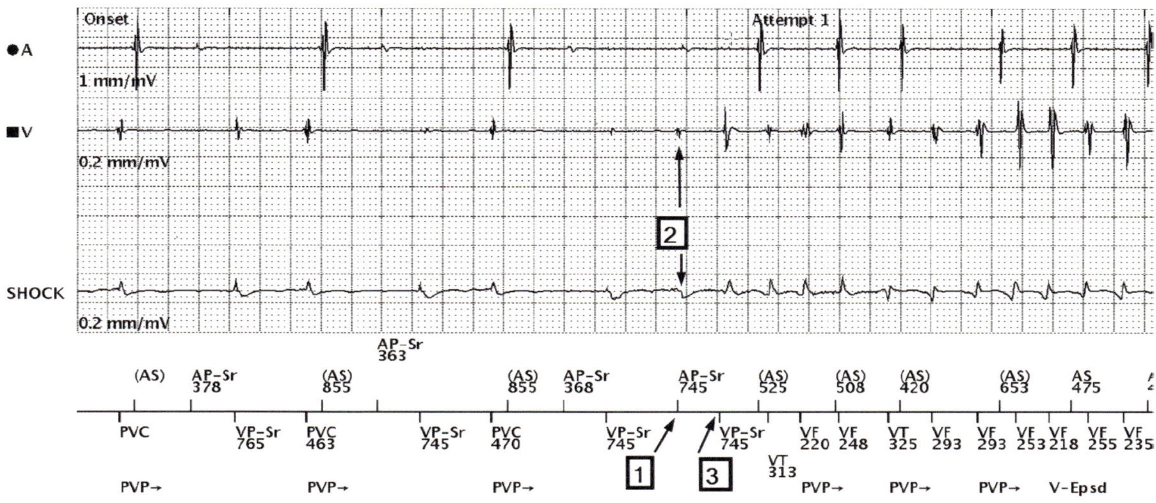

Figure 48a.

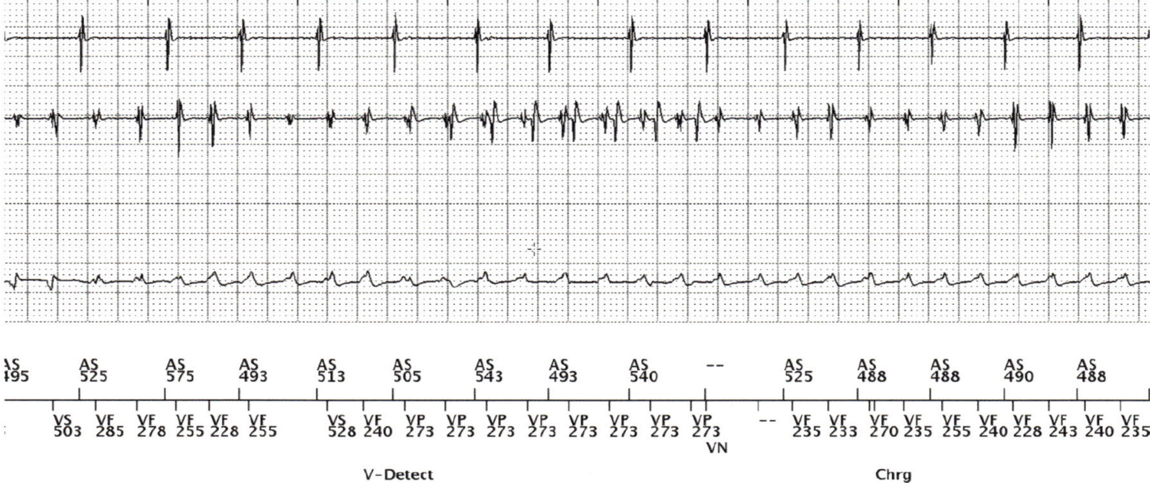

Figure 48b.

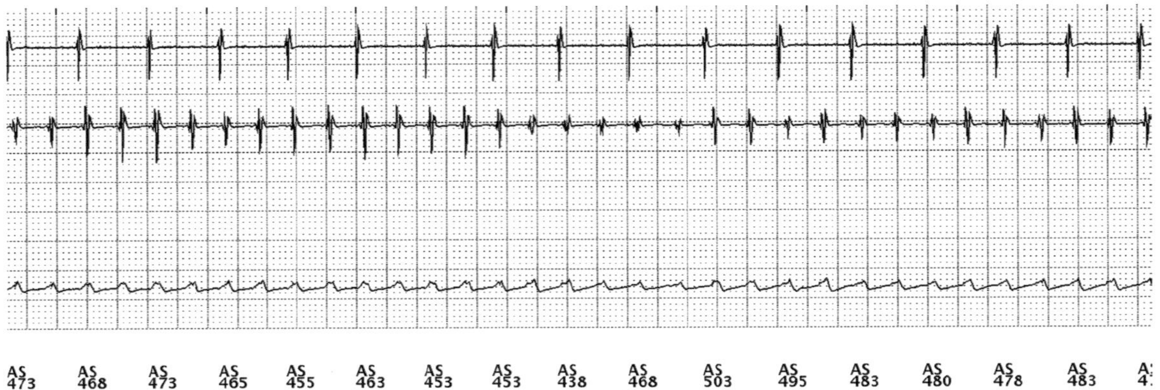

Figure 48c.

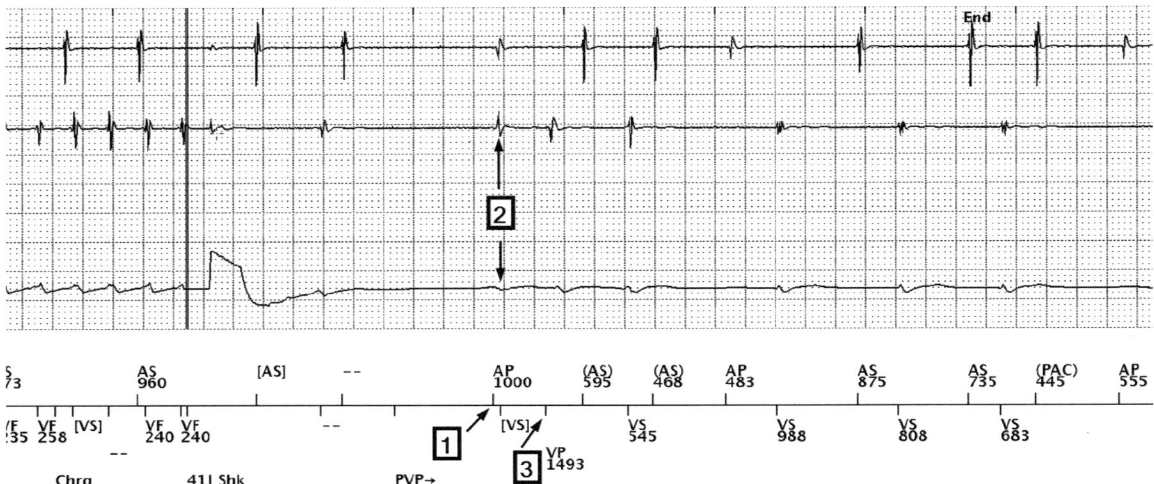

Figure 48d.

Brady	
Normal Settings	
Mode	DDDR
Lower Rate Limit	60 ppm
Maximum Tracking Rate	140 ppm
Maximum Sensor Rate	140 ppm
Paced AV Delay	180 - 350 ms
Sensed AV Delay	180 - 350 ms
A-Refractory (PVARP)	240 - 310 ms
V-Refractory (VRP)	210 - 250 ms
PVARP after PVC	400 ms
AV Search +	Off
Blanking	
A-Blank after V-Pace	Smart ms
A-Blank after V-Sense	Smart ms
V-Blank after A-Pace	65 ms
Noise Response	DOO
Rate Enhancements	
Rate Smoothing	
Up	Off %
Down	Off %

Figure 48e.

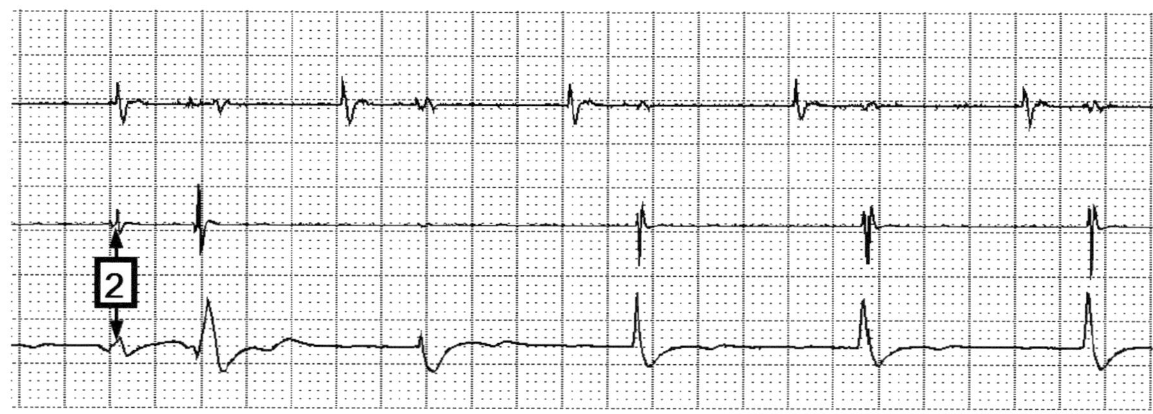
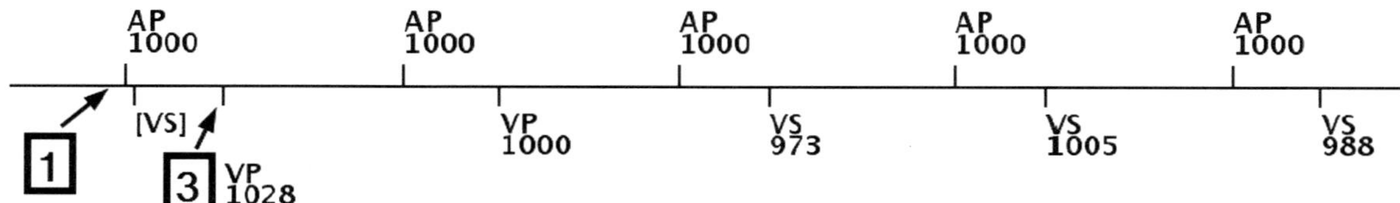

Figure 48f.

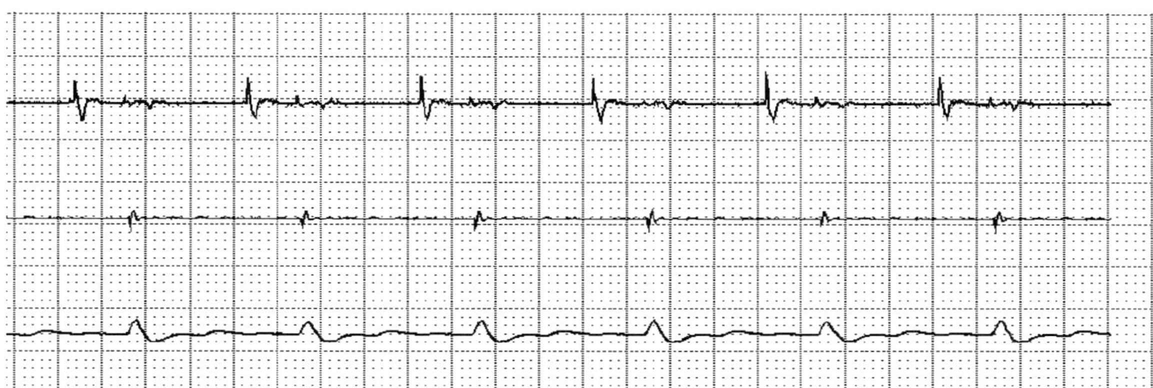
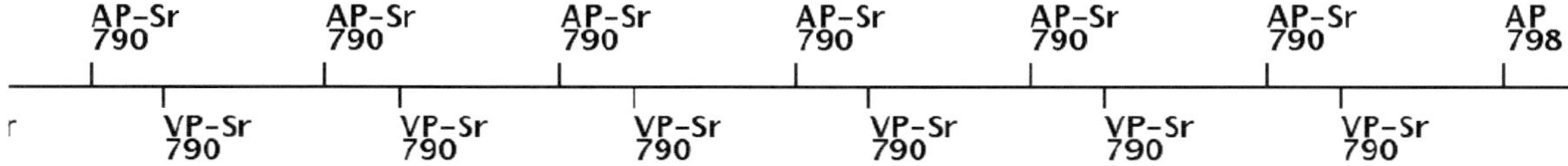

Figure 48g.

ANALYSIS

1. In Figure 48a, there is atrial pacing impulse at sensor driven rate [1] followed by a PVC [2] that falls within the V-Blank after A-Pace period of 65 ms (see settings in Figure 48e). Following the atrial pace, once the AV interval expires, the device delivers a ventricular pacing impulse which occurs in the vulnerable period and unfortunately led to the episode seen here. Boston Scientific devices do not have safety pacing, but they have a retriggerable noise window. Pacing occurs when the AV delay expires and when noise is sensed in the noise window.

2. In Figure 48d, one 41-J shock converts the arrhythmia. Shortly after this, we see the same sequence of events that precipitated this episode; an atrial pace [1] followed by a blanked PVC [2], and a ventricular pacing impulse [3] delivered in or near the vulnerable period.

3. The EGM in Figure 48f was obtained when the patient was seen at the hospital bedside where the same sequence of events, [1], [2], and [3], recurred. The V-Blank after A-Pace period of 65 ms can be programmed to the SMART setting, which promotes sensing of PVCs by shortening the cross-chamber blanking period to 35 ms following an A-paced event and 15 ms following an A-sensed event. However, because other episodes occurred that were initiated by PVCs, an attempt to suppress the occurrence of PVCs was made by increasing the lower rate limit from 60 to 70 bpm and shortening the maximum AV delays to 240 ms. As seen in Figure 48g, this dramatically reduced the frequency of PVCs.

CLINICAL RESPONSE

Pacing in the vulnerable period during repolarization can lead to ventricular arrhythmias. Functional undersensing of ventricular events during blanking period following an atrial events can lead to ventricular pacing in the vulnerable period. Changing the lower rate and shortening the blanking periods helped with avoiding these pacing-related arrhythmias.

49 | Ventricular Pacing in the Vulnerable Period During Atrial Flutter

DEVICE: Boston Scientific Inogen X4 G148 CRT-D

PATIENT: A 72-year-old male recently implanted with a LVAD. The device nurse specialist was called to see the patient due to ventricular pacing artifacts on ECG monitor in what appears to be the vulnerable period of QRS complexes. The EGM is shown in **Figure 49a** and programmed parameters are shown in **Figure 49b**. What is the cause of abnormality described?

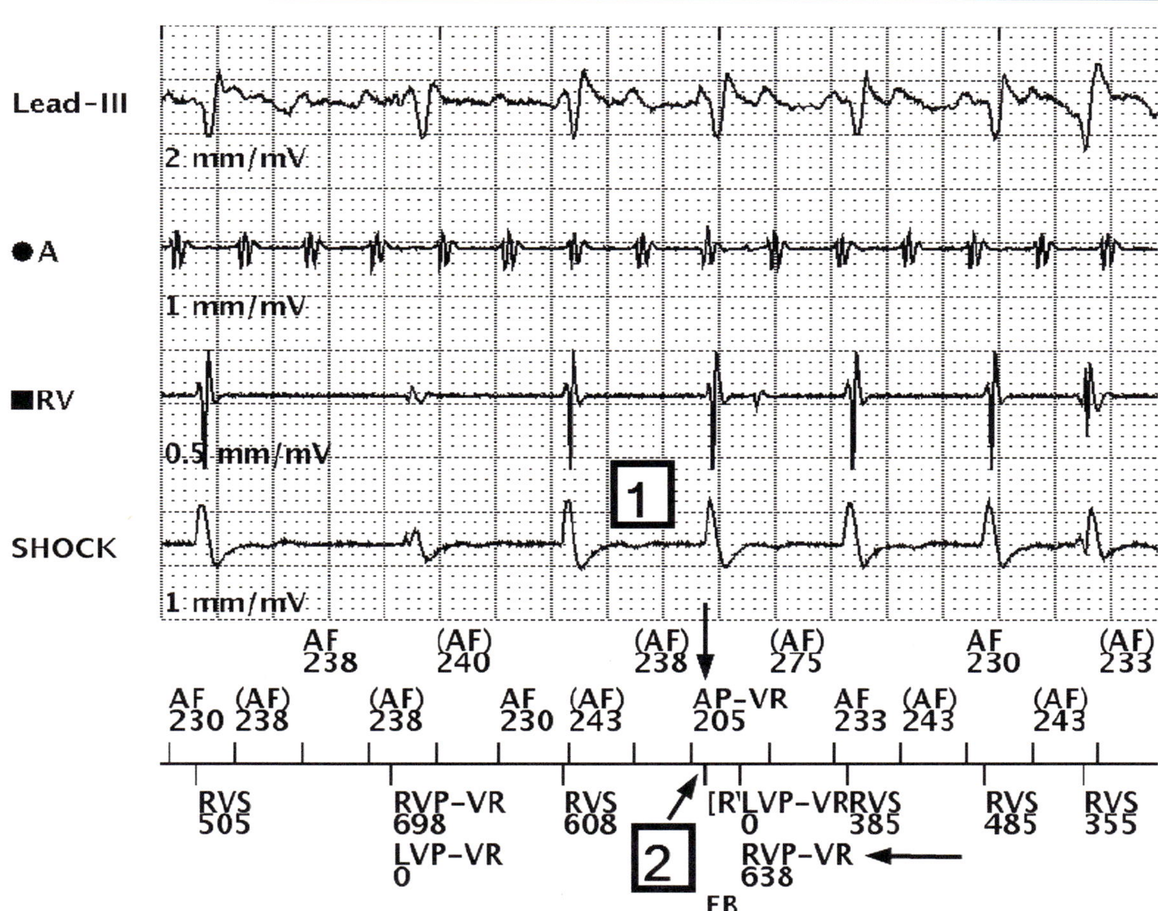

Figure 49a.

Brady/CRT	
Normal Settings	
Mode	DDD
Lower Rate Limit	90 ppm
Maximum Tracking Rate	130 ppm
Maximum Sensor Rate	130 ppm
Paced AV Delay	150 - 180 ms
Sensed AV Delay	125 - 150 ms
A-Refractory (PVARP)	180 - 340 ms
RV-Refractory (RVRP)	180 - 340 ms
LV-Refractory (LVRP)	250 ms

Atrial Tachy	
Therapy	
ATR Mode Switch Details	
ATR Mode Switch	On
Trigger Rate	150 bpm
Duration	8 cycles
Entry Count	8 cycles
Exit Count	8 cycles
Fallback	
Mode	[3] DDIR
Time	00:30 mm:ss
ATR/VTR Fallback LRL	90 ppm
Ventricular Rate Regulation	Min

Figure 49b.

ANALYSIS

1. In this episode, atrial flutter waves consistently fall into the postventricular atrial refractory period (PVARP) [1]. Despite ongoing atrial flutter, inappropriate atrial pacing occurs (see down arrows ↓) due to flutter waves falling into the refractory period.

2. For this patient with conducted atrial flutter, V-sensed events fall into RV blanking after A-Pace [2]. When this occurs, once the AV interval expires, the device delivers a V-pacing artifact following the intrinsic QRS, which may fall in the vulnerable period of repolarization (see left arrows ←), putting the patient at risk for ventricular arrhythmia.

CLINICAL RESPONSE

By changing the Fallback mode, which was programmed DDIR [3], to one that eliminates atrial pacing, such as VDIR, the potential for blanked ventricular events and subsequent V-pacing during the vulnerable period was also eliminated (**Figure 49c**).

AF) 90
AF 235
AF 233
AF 235
(AF) 243
AF 238
(AF) 243
AF 233
(AF) 245
(AF) 245
(AF) 238
(AF) 235
AF 230
(AF) 238
(AF) 235
RVS 503
RVS 503
RVS 605
RVP–VR 620
LVP–VR 0
RVS 568
RVS 508

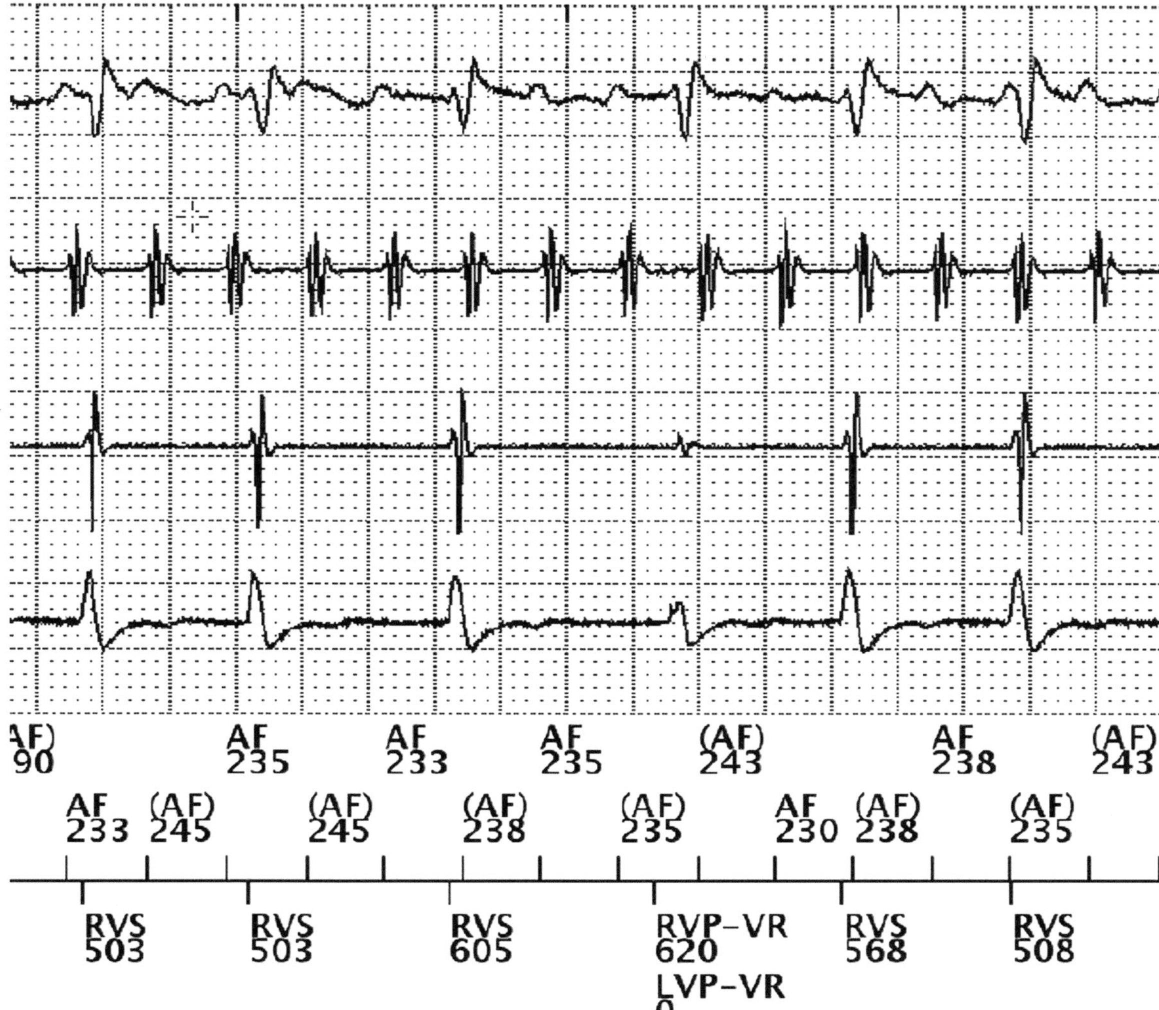

Figure 49c.

50 | T-Wave Oversensing

DEVICE: St. Jude Medical* Unify Assura 3357-40C CRT-D

PATIENT: A 28-year-old patient with hypoplastic left heart syndrome and previous Fontan procedure has an abdominally placed CRT-D with an epicardial lead system. The LV lead is programmed off due to chronic failure to capture. Routine remote follow-up reported non-sustained RV oversensing episodes as shown in **Figure 50a**.

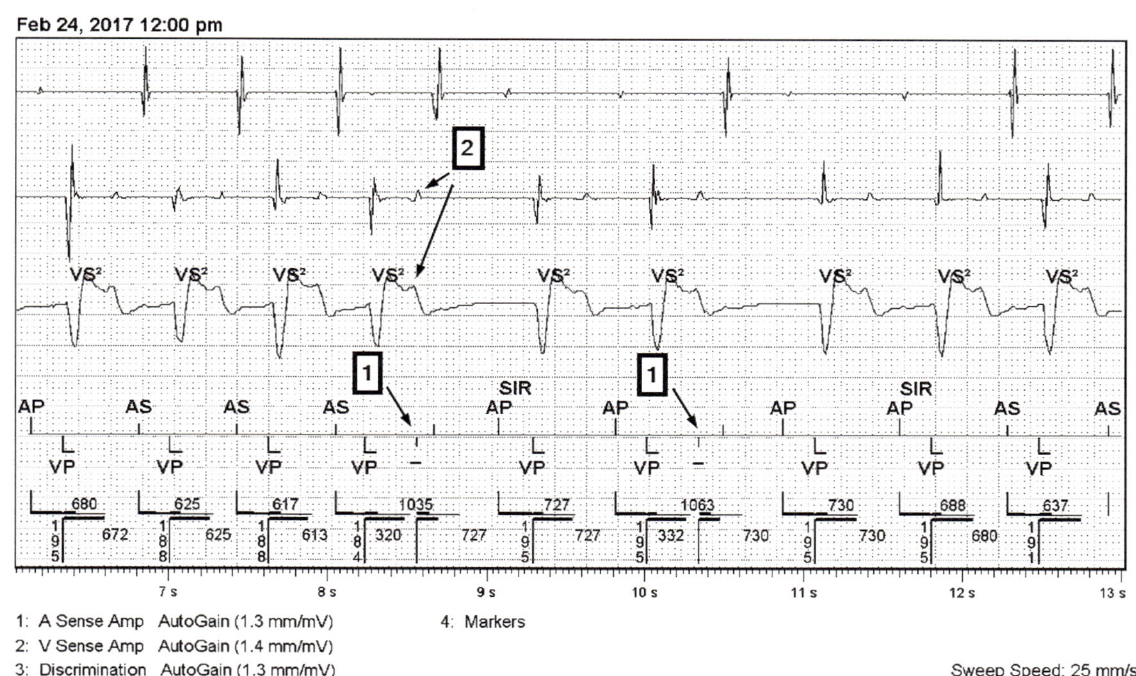

Figure 50a.

ANALYSIS

1. In this EGM example, the device is intermittently double counting some of the ventricular paced complexes. The ventricular sensed events on the V sense amplifier following the VP meet the VT detection rate criteria [1]. The manufacturer's " – " channel marker indicates an unbinned event, as the current interval and the average interval do not match. The intrinsic atrial events following the double count fall in the refractory period and is not tracked resulting in loss of AV synchrony. Due to oversensing of T waves and subsequent "A" functional undersensing, we see intermittent pauses between QRS complexes on the far-field ECG (discrimination).

---

*St. Jude Medical is now Abbott.

2. It appears that T waves are intermittently oversensed following ventricular pacing. Deflections are observed on both the V sense amplifier EGM and discrimination EGM [2]. But only the V sense amplifier is double counting, the discrimination channel counts one event. This results in a mismatch between the V sense amplifier and the discrimination counters.

CLINICAL RESPONSE

The nonsustained RV oversensing feature (NSRVO) on St. Jude Medical ICDs is a noise-discrimination algorithm designed to minimize the potential for inappropriate therapies due to oversensing or other failure mechanisms. When a high ventricular rate signal is sensed on the near-field ventricular sense amplifier the algorithm compares that rate to the sensed signal on the far-field discrimination channel. If there is a mismatch in these two channels, the NSRVO is indicated. The T-wave deflection [2] is not sensed on the discrimination channel. This episode is classified as nonsustained RV oversensing and prevents the device from progressing to detection and therapy. These episodes require further investigation to verify the NSRVO discrimination is appropriate. It is important to contact Abbott/St. Jude technical services for review and programming recommendations. Technical services confirmed T-wave oversensing and suggested changing the Post-Paced Decay Delay from 0 ms to 95 ms, and changing the Post-Paced Threshold Start from 1.0 mV to 1.1 mV (**Figures 50b** and **50c**). These changes eliminated T-wave oversensing and allowed appropriate tracking of the intrinsic atrial rhythm.

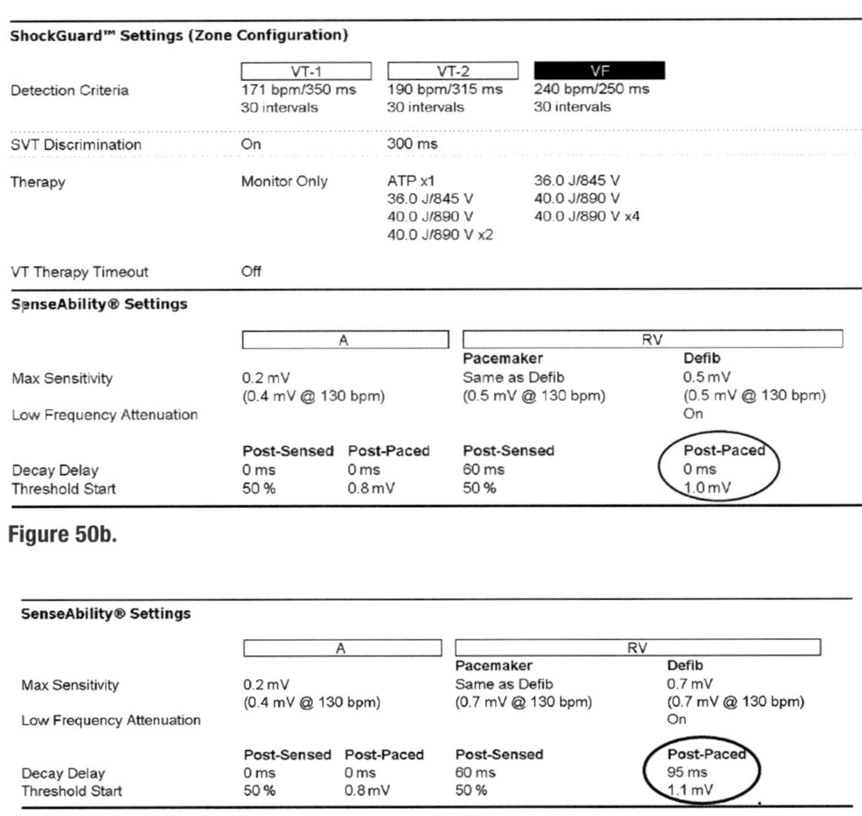

ShockGuard™ Settings (Zone Configuration)

	VT-1	VT-2	VF
Detection Criteria	171 bpm/350 ms 30 intervals	190 bpm/315 ms 30 intervals	240 bpm/250 ms 30 intervals
SVT Discrimination	On	300 ms	
Therapy	Monitor Only	ATP x1 36.0 J/845 V 40.0 J/890 V 40.0 J/890 V x2	36.0 J/845 V 40.0 J/890 V 40.0 J/890 V x4
VT Therapy Timeout	Off		

SenseAbility® Settings

	A		RV	
			Pacemaker	Defib
Max Sensitivity	0.2 mV (0.4 mV @ 130 bpm)		Same as Defib (0.5 mV @ 130 bpm)	0.5 mV (0.5 mV @ 130 bpm)
Low Frequency Attenuation				On
	Post-Sensed	Post-Paced	Post-Sensed	Post-Paced
Decay Delay	0 ms	0 ms	60 ms	0 ms
Threshold Start	50 %	0.8 mV	50 %	1.0 mV

Figure 50b.

SenseAbility® Settings

	A		RV	
			Pacemaker	Defib
Max Sensitivity	0.2 mV (0.4 mV @ 130 bpm)		Same as Defib (0.7 mV @ 130 bpm)	0.7 mV (0.7 mV @ 130 bpm)
Low Frequency Attenuation				On
	Post-Sensed	Post-Paced	Post-Sensed	Post-Paced
Decay Delay	0 ms	0 ms	60 ms	95 ms
Threshold Start	50 %	0.8 mV	50 %	1.1 mV

Figure 50c.

51 | RV Lead Integrity Warning and T-Wave Oversensing Discrimination

DEVICE: Medtronic Evera XT DR DDMB1D4 DC ICD

PATIENT: A 56-year-old patient with hypertrophic nonobstructive cardiomyopathy had experienced two syncopal episodes during exercise. Ambulatory monitoring demonstrated non-sustained ventricular tachycardia, and the patient was implanted with a dual-chamber ICD for primary prevention. A remote alert transmission was received due to an RV lead integrity warning. The RV lead warning alerts us to a different problem. Consider the following messages (**Figure 51a**) from the remote transmission. What was the reason for the warning alert?

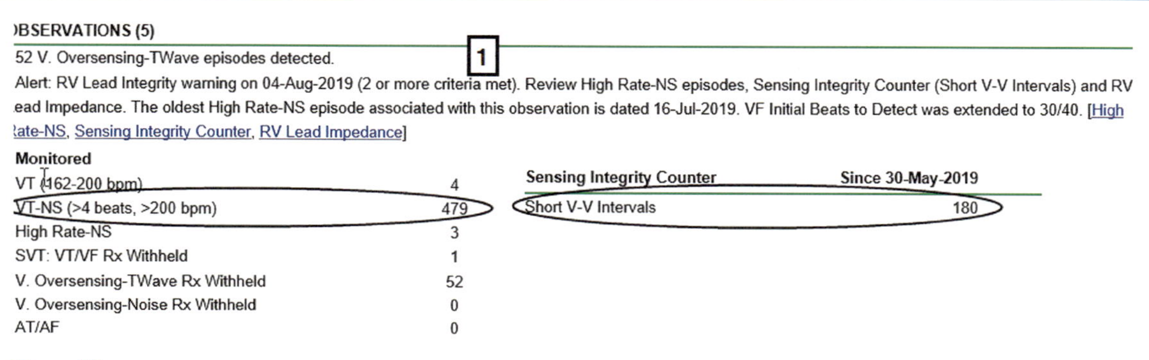

Figure 51a.

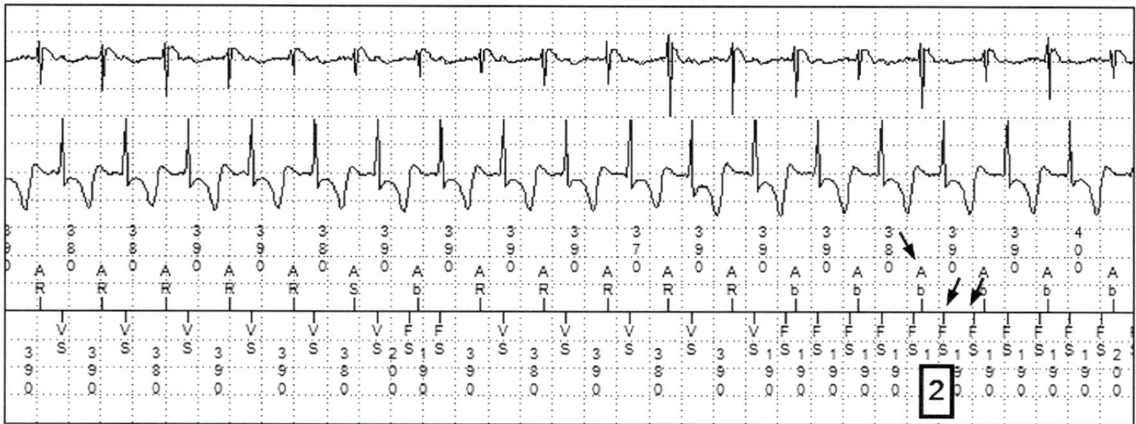

Figure 51b.

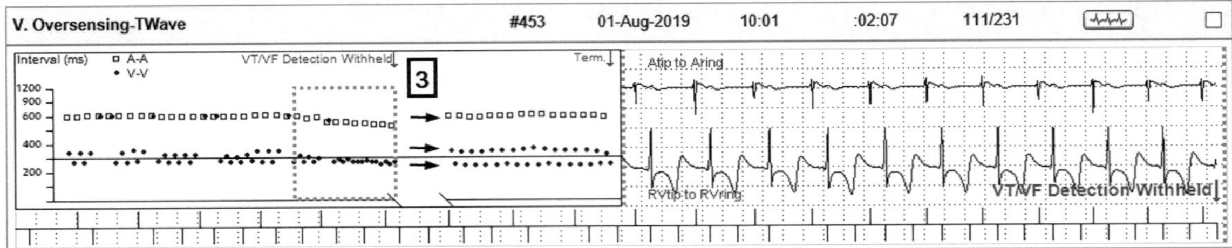

Figure 51c.

ANALYSIS

1. The RV lead integrity alert [1] monitors the frequency of rapid, nonsustained VT episodes, frequency of short ventricular intervals on the Sensing Integrity Counter (SIC), and RV pacing lead impedance measurements. If two of the three criteria are met, the device issues an alert notification and reprograms tachycardia detection to 30 of 40 intervals. Detection prolongation reduces the risk of inappropriate therapy. In this specific case, fast NSVT and SIC triggered the RV lead integrity alert.

2. The RV lead integrity alerts us to a problem, but the real issue is something different. The EGM in **Figure 51b** demonstrates that the fast NSVT and SIC are actually the result of T-wave oversensing [2]. The double-counting of ventricular events is evident and leads to inappropriate detection of ventricular arrhythmia.

VT/VF Detection

		V. Interval (Rate)	Initial	Redetect
VF	On	300 ms (200 bpm)	30/40	12/16
FVT	OFF			
VT	OFF	360 ms (167 bpm)	16	12
Monitor	Monitor	370 ms (162 bpm)	32	

PR Logic/Wavelet		Other Enhancements		Sensitivity	
AF/Afl	On	Stability	Off	Atrial	0.30 mV
Sinus Tach	On	Onset	Off	RV	0.30 mV
Other 1:1 SVTs	Off	High Rate Timeout			
Wavelet	On	VF Zone Only	Off		
Template	29-May-2019	TWave	On		
Match Threshold	70 %	RV Lead Noise	On+Timeout		
Auto Collection	On	Timeout	0.75 min		
SVT V. Limit	260 ms				

Figure 51d.

3. The episode plot and the EGM in **Figure 51c** show T-wave oversensing with the signature pattern of two ventricular events for every atrial event. This pattern is often described as train tracks on the interval plot. The interval from R to the T wave is often shorter than T to next R wave, resulting in alternation of short and long intervals. Fortunately, the T-wave discrimination feature (**Figure 51d**) of this device appropriately recognized the signature of T-wave oversensing and withheld delivery of inappropriate therapy [3]. The T-wave discrimination feature detects the morphological differences in the alternating R and T waves. R waves typically have higher-frequency content than T waves. The algorithm uses this data to distinguish the R- and T-wave patterns from a true ventricular arrhythmia.

CLINICAL RESPONSE

The patient was assessed in the clinic. The T-wave oversensing events correlated with patient exercise. The patient's heart rate routinely increases to 160 bpm during exercise. Medtronic technical support was consulted and recommended changing the RV sensitivity from 0.3 mV to 0.45 mV (Figure 51d). The patient exercised in the clinic, and no T-wave oversensing was observed. The patient subsequently followed his routine intense exercise workout, and his device was reassessed with no T-wave oversensing observed. Inappropriate therapies due to T-wave oversensing can be tackled by increasing the detection rate, changing the sensitivity, changing the sensing vector (bipolar or integrated bipolar) or by use of special algorithms.

52 | Subcutaneous ICD Oversensing

DEVICE: Boston Scientific Emblem A209 S-ICD

PATIENT: A 52-year-old patient with a history of hypertrophic obstructive cardiomyopathy has undergone septal myectomy. The patient also has a family history of sudden cardiac death, and the decision is made for implantation of a subcutaneous ICD. A routine remote follow-up includes an alert for an untreated episode. Consider the EGM excerpts in **Figure 52a** from the remote transmission episode. Device parameter settings are in **Figure 52b**.

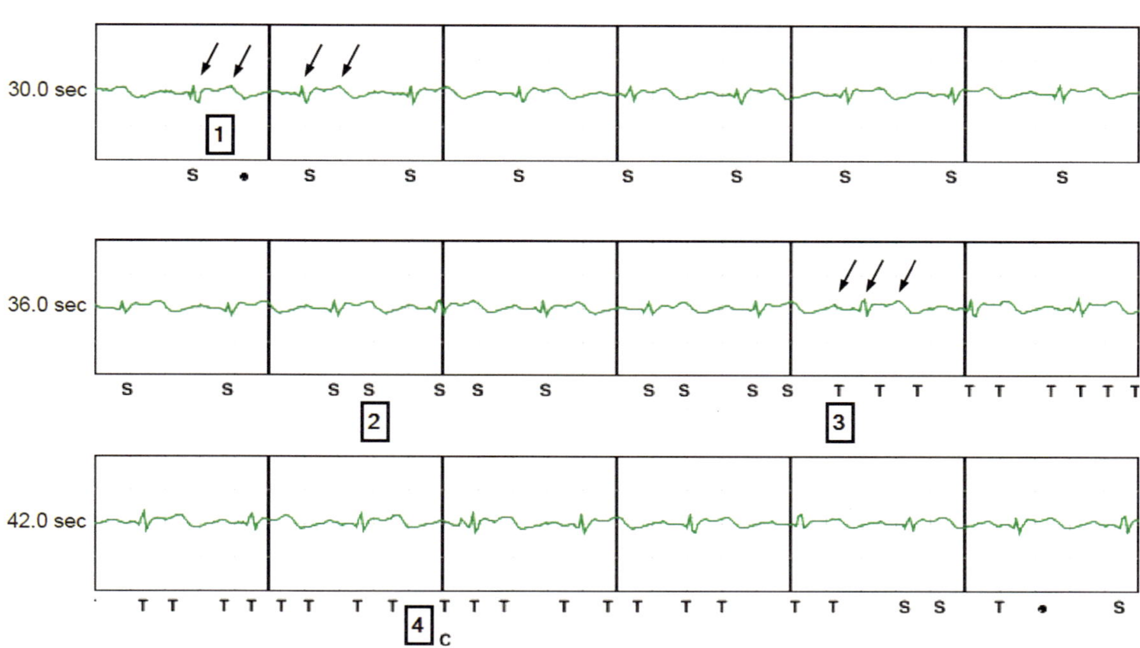

Figure 52a.

Tachy Therapy Settings	
Therapy	ON
Shock Zone	220 bpm
Conditional Shock Zone	200 bpm
Additional Device Settings	
Post Shock Pacing	ON
Gain Setting	1X
Sensing Configuration	Alternate
SMART Pass	OFF

S = Sense
P = Pace
N = Noise
T = Tachy Detection
C = Charge Start
E = Charge End
• = Discard
♥ = Event End

Figure 52b.

1. The first fast detected interval falls into the Conditional Shock Zone at 200 bpm (300 ms). In the Conditional zone, the device uses a Certification Phase algorithm to help discriminate accurate heart rate from noise events or double-counting of single cardiac events. The EGM waveform suggests normal sinus rhythm and not true arrhythmia. This first fast interval [1] appears to be T-wave oversensing and is counted but is appropriately labeled with the "discard" channel marker by the device algorithm (• = Discard). The following QRS complex is sensed appropriately without T-wave oversensing (S = Sense).

2. The intermittent oversensing of T waves persists [2]. These events are now recognized as sensed events and are therefore counted by the Certification Phase algorithm toward meeting criteria for tachycardia counters.

3. The device begins to triple sense the PQRST complex [3]. The R-to-R average now falls into detection as treatable intervals, and the device begins a moving window of 24 certified events. If 18 of 24 intervals are found to be treatable the device begins capacitor charging.

4. The 18 of 24 criteria is met, and the device begins charging [4]. The 18 of 24 criteria continues during charging. The oversensed events become more intermittent, and the R-to-R average drops out of the detection zones.

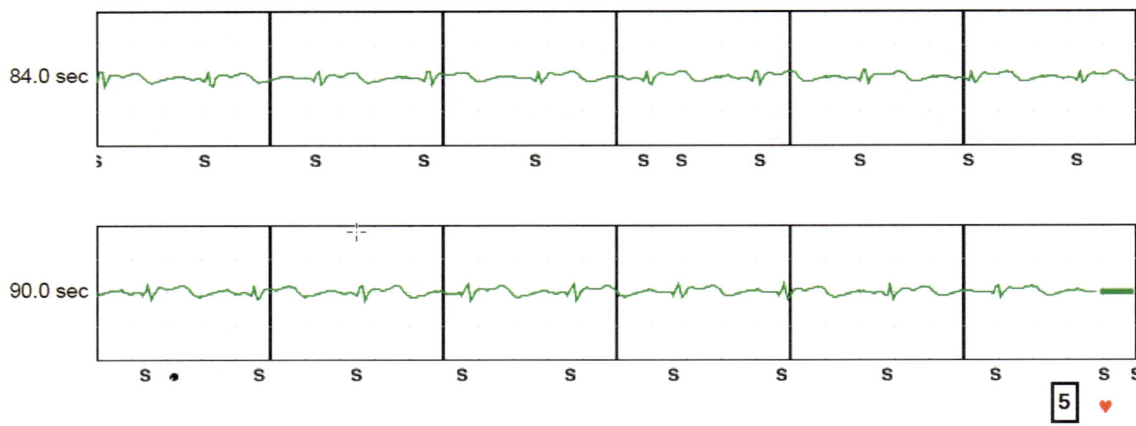

Figure 52c.

5. As the episode continues the oversensing markedly decreases as shown in **Figure 52c**. When the R-to-R average interval becomes longer than the conditional zone plus 40 ms (300 ms + 40 ms = 340 ms) therapy delivery is aborted, and the episode is declared untreated. The "heart" channel marker indicates the end of the event [5].

The findings were reviewed with the electrophysiologist and confirmed as inappropriate oversensing and not true arrhythmia. The patient was contacted, and arrangements were made for the patient to be seen. When the patient was seen in clinic, the primary sensing vector was changed from alternate (distal electrode ring to can) to primary (proximal electrode ring to can). The patient underwent provocative maneuvers, and exercise tests without any oversensing detected using the primary vector. The SMART pass filter was also turned on to prevent T-wave oversensing. The algorithm works by reducing low-frequency signals of the T waves from a sensed electrogram, thereby reducing the chance of oversensing. The patient will continue to be monitored with routine remote follow-up.

53 | Mode Switch During VT Detection

FIRST OF TWO EXAMPLES

DEVICE: St. Jude Medical* Quadra Assura 3369-40Q CRT-D

PATIENT: A 66-year-old male was implanted with a BiV device for ischemic cardiomyopathy. Later that year, the patient underwent implantation of a LVAD, at which time ventricular pacing was programmed to RV Only. The EGMs (**Figures 53a**, **53b**, **53c**, and **53d**) and programmed parameters (**Figure 53e**) are shown below.

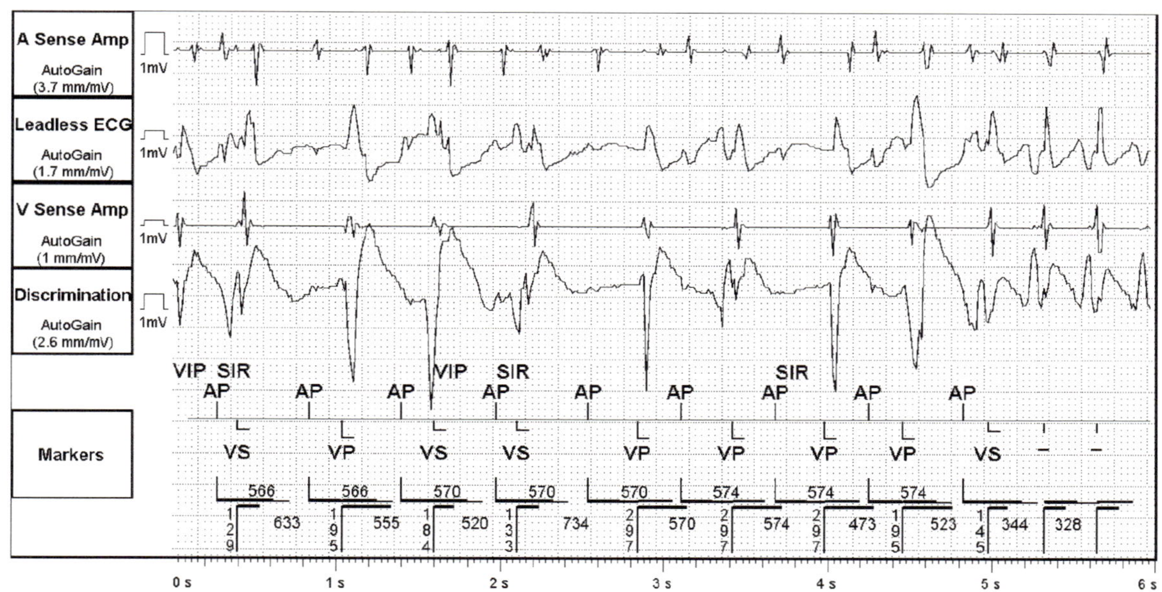

Figure 53a.

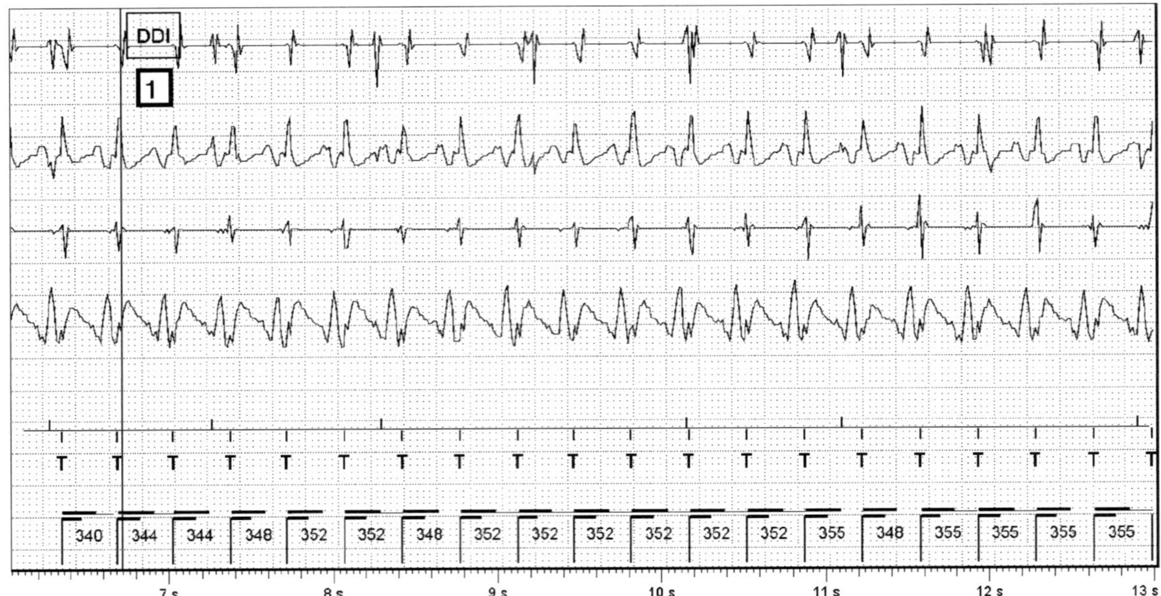

Figure 53b.

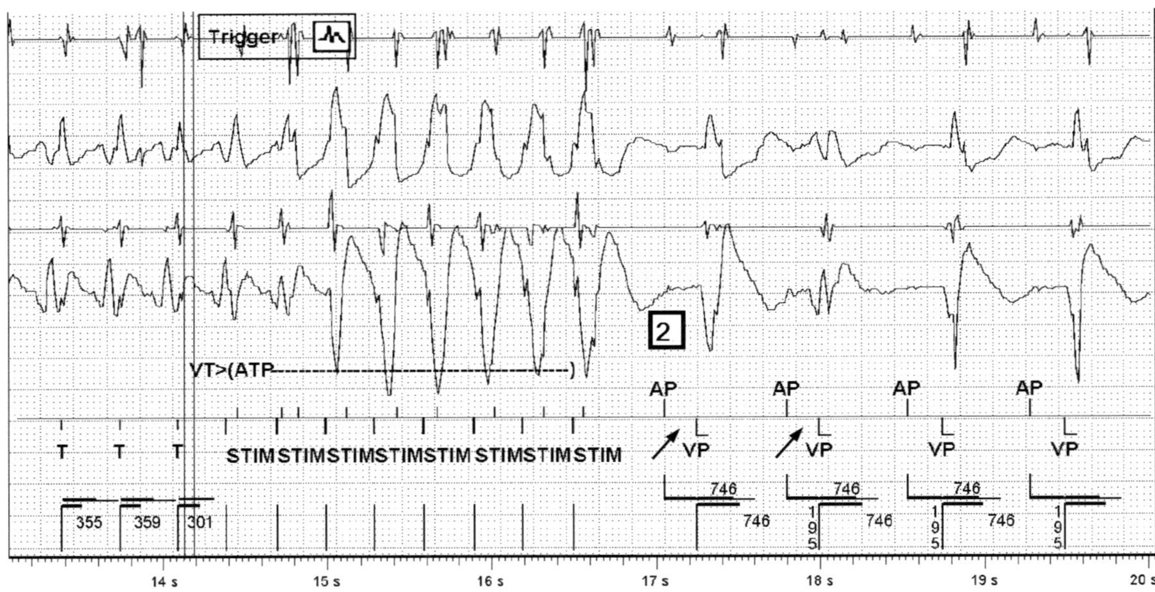

Figure 53c.

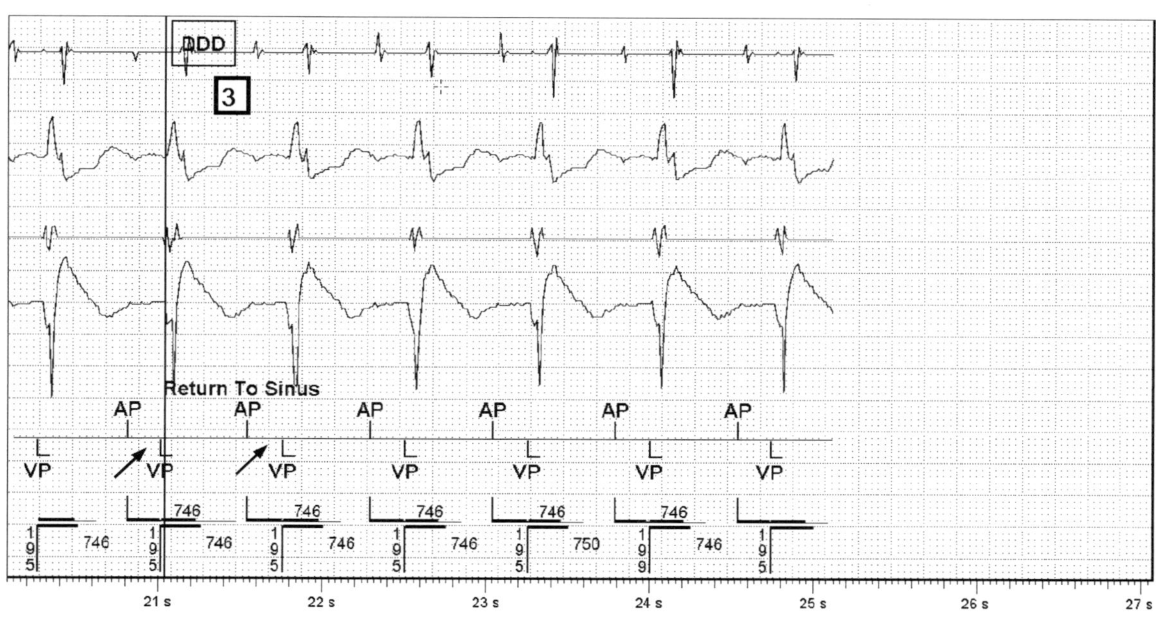

Figure 53d.

Basic Operation

Mode	DDDR
Ventricular Pacing	RV Only
V. Triggering	Off
Magnet Response	Normal
V. Noise Reversion Mode	VOO
Episodal Pacing Mode	DDI
Sensor	On
Threshold (Measured Avg.)	Auto (-0.5) (2.0)
Slope	8
Max Sensor Rate	120 bpm
Reaction Time	Fast
Recovery Time	Medium

Rates

Base Rate	80 bpm
Rest Rate	Off
Max Sensor Rate	120 bpm
Max Track Rate	115 bpm
Hysteresis Rate	Off
2:1 Block Rate	120 bpm

Delays

Paced AV Delay	200 ms
Sensed AV Delay	200 ms

Redetection & Post-Detection

VT Redetection	6 intervals
Sinus Redetection	Nominal (5 intervals)
Post VF Detection	Same as VT
Post VT Detection	Same as VT

ShockGuard™ Settings (Zone Configuration)

	VT	VF
Detection Criteria	150 bpm/400 ms 24 intervals	200 bpm/300 ms 12 intervals
SVT Discrimination	On	
Therapy	ATP x3 30.0 J/791 V 38.0 J/890 V 38.0 J/890 V x2	ATP x1 30.0 J/791 V 38.0 J/890 V 38.0 J/890 V x4
VT Therapy Timeout	Off	

ATP Details

ATP Pulse Amplitude	7.5 V
ATP Pulse Width	1.0 ms

	VT		VF
	Therapy 1	**Therapy 2**	**Therapy 1**
ATP Type			ATP While Charging
ATP Upper Rate Cutoff			250 bpm/240 ms
Number of Bursts	3		1
Number of Stimuli	8		8
Add Stimuli per Burst	Off		
Burst Cycle Length	85 %		85 %
Min. Burst Cycle Length	200 ms		170 ms
Readaptive	Off		
Scanning	On (Dec)		
Scan Step	10 ms		
Ramp	Off		Off

Figure 53e.

ANALYSIS EXAMPLE 1

1. In Figures 53a and 53b, following the third non-sinus interval, the device declares an episode and switches to the Episodal Pacing Mode [1] which, for this patient, is DDI.

2. Following delivery of Antitachycardia Pacing (ATP) and successful conversion to sinus rhythm, the patient is AV-paced at the lower rate limit of 80 bpm with a paced AV delay of 200 ms, as programmed. See [2] in Figure 53c. In this case, no unwanted effects to the patient's rhythm occur.

3. Once the device has detected an arrhythmia, the sinus redetection parameter determines the number of sinus intervals needed in order for the device to declare the end of the episode and return to a tracking mode such as DDD. See [3] in Figure 53d.

SECOND OF TWO EXAMPLES

DEVICE: St. Jude Medical* Unify Assura 3357-40 CRT-D

PATIENT: A 71-year-old male with a history of paroxysmal atrial fibrillation, right heart failure and dilated cardiomyopathy was implanted with a BiV device. The EGMs (**Figures 53f, 53g, 53h,** and **53i**) and programmed parameters (**Figure 53j**) are shown below.

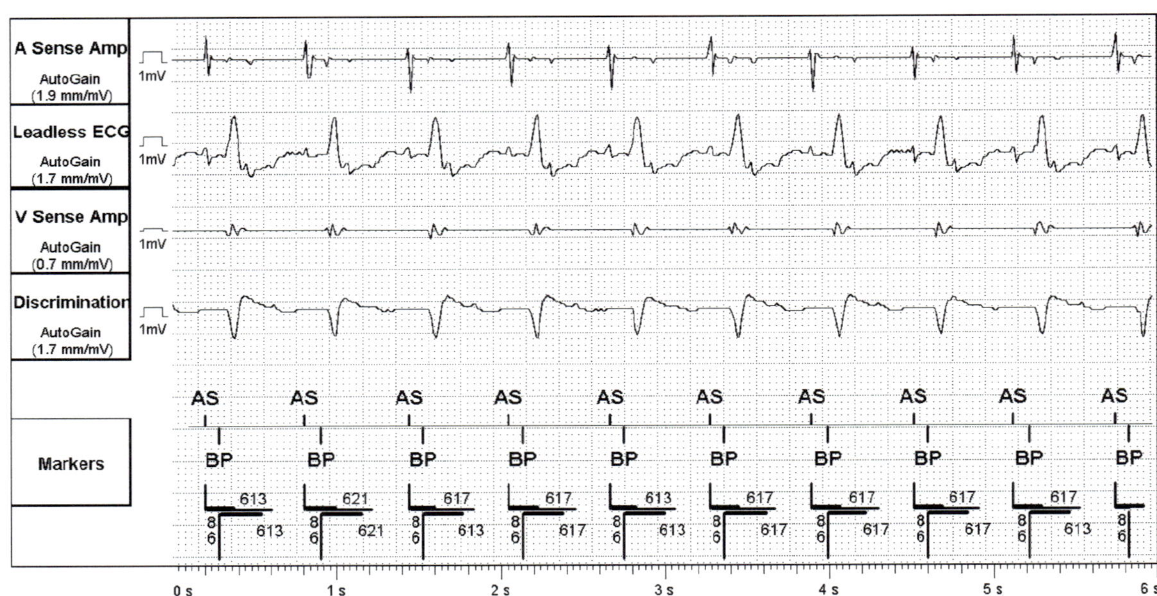

Figure 53f.

---

*St. Jude Medical is now Abbott.

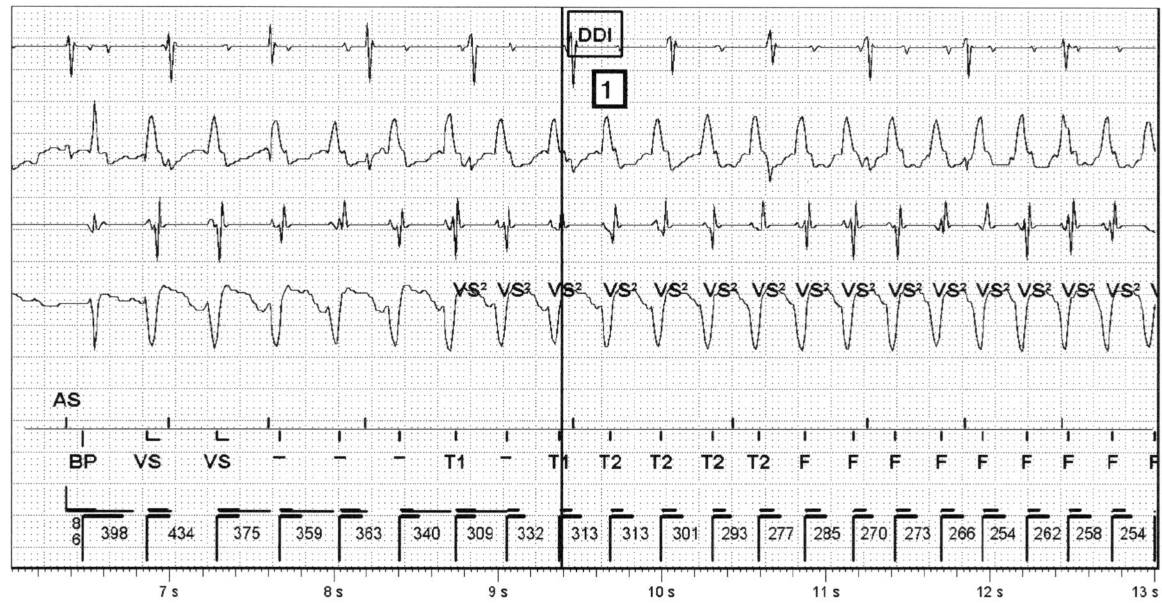

Figure 53g.

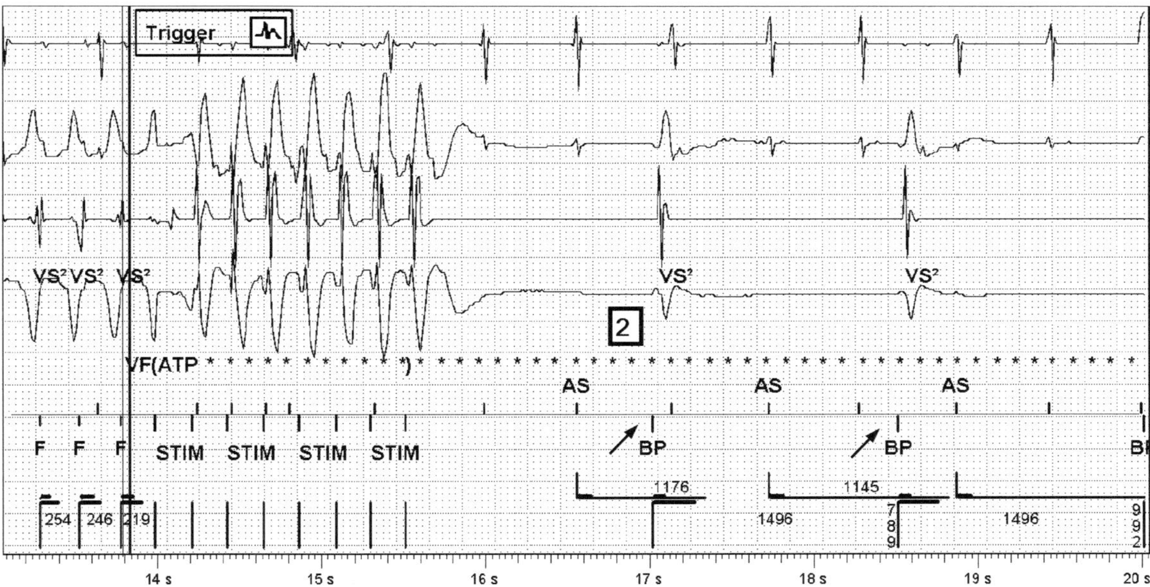

Figure 53h.

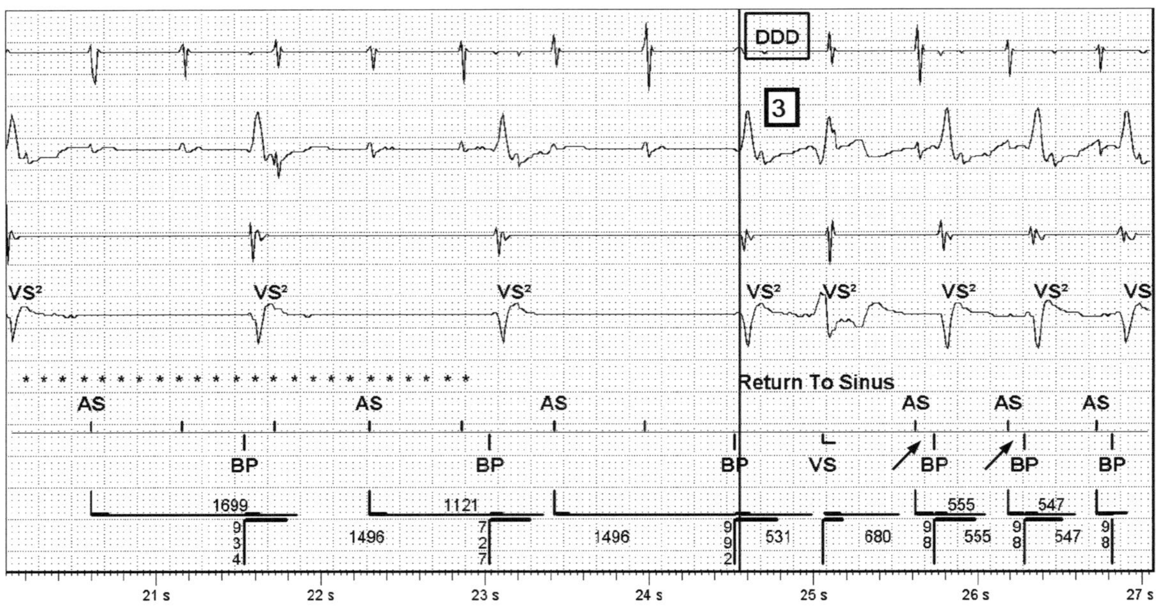

Figure 53i.

Basic Operation	
Mode	DDD
Ventricular Pacing	Simul.
V. Triggering	Off
Magnet Response	Normal
V. Noise Reversion Mode	DOO
Episodal Pacing Mode	DDI
Sensor	Passive
Threshold (Measured Avg.)	Auto (+0.0) (2.0)
Slope	8
Max Sensor Rate	120 bpm
Reaction Time	Fast
Recovery Time	Medium

Rates	
Base Rate	40 bpm
Rest Rate	Off
Max Sensor Rate	120 bpm
Max Track Rate	140 bpm
Hysteresis Rate	Off
2:1 Block Rate	170 bpm

Delays	
Paced AV Delay	130 ms
Sensed AV Delay	100 ms

Redetection & Post-Detection	
VT Redetection	6 intervals
Sinus Redetection	Nominal (5 intervals)
Post VF/VT-2 Detection	Same as VT-2

ShockGuard™ Settings (Zone Configuration)

	VT-1	VT-2	VF
Detection Criteria	160 bpm/375 ms 30 intervals	184 bpm/325 ms 12 intervals	206 bpm/290 ms 12 intervals
SVT Discrimination	Off	Off	
Therapy	Monitor Only	ATP x1 36.0 J/845 V 40.0 J/890 V 40.0 J/890 V x2	ATP x1 36.0 J/845 V 40.0 J/890 V 40.0 J/890 V x4
VT Therapy Timeout	Off		

ATP Details

ATP Pulse Amplitude	7.5 V	
ATP Pulse Width	1.0 ms	

	VT-2		VF
	Therapy 1	Therapy 2	Therapy 1
ATP Type			ATP While Charging
ATP Upper Rate Cutoff			250 bpm/240 ms
Number of Bursts	1		1
Number of Stimuli	8		8
Burst Cycle Length	88 %		88 %
Min. Burst Cycle Length	200 ms		170 ms
Scan Step	10 ms		
Ramp	Off		Off

Figure 53j.

1. Following what the pulse generator recognizes as the third non-sinus interval, there is a mode switch to the programmed Episodal Pacing Mode of DDI. See [1] in Figure 53g.

2. After delivery of ATP and successful conversion to sinus rhythm, the device maintains the Episodal Pacing Mode of DDI leaving this patient with a loss of AV synchrony, due to an intact sinus node and the temporary nontracking mode of DDI. See [2] in Figure 53h. In this case, there is a sinus rate of 100 bpm combined with a programmed ventricular base pacing rate of 40 bpm.

3. When the device redetects sinus rhythm per the programmed sinus redetection requirement of five intervals, it returns to a tracking mode and AV synchrony is restored. See [3] in Figure 53i.

CLINICAL RESPONSE

For patients such as the one in Example 1, with a sinus rate below the lower rate limit leading to atrial pacing followed by ventricular pacing once the programmed paced AV delay has expired, the nontracking mode has no negative effect. In Example 2, while the loss of AV synchrony is brief, one might consider increasing the lower rate limit to 60 bpm to provide a more normal heartrate. However, AV synchrony will not be restored until redetection of sinus rhythm, as the available options for the Episodal Pacing Mode include only the nontracking modes of DDI, VVI, and AAI.

54 | Single-Chamber ICD with Atrial Sensing

DEVICE: Biotronik Lumax 740 VR-T DX SC ICD

PATIENT: A 62-year-old patient with ischemic cardiomyopathy was implanted for primary prevention with a Biotronik single-chamber, single-lead ICD with atrial sensing capability. Biotronik's DX lead technology incorporates two additional electrodes on the RV lead. These electrodes form a floating dipole (cathode ring and anode ring) in the atrium that allows for atrial sensing. This feature provides atrial diagnostics and dual-chamber discrimination within a single RV lead. Consider the following EGMs (**Figure 54a** and **Figure 54c**) from routine, remote follow-up. Atrial sensing programmed parameters are shown in **Figure 54b**.

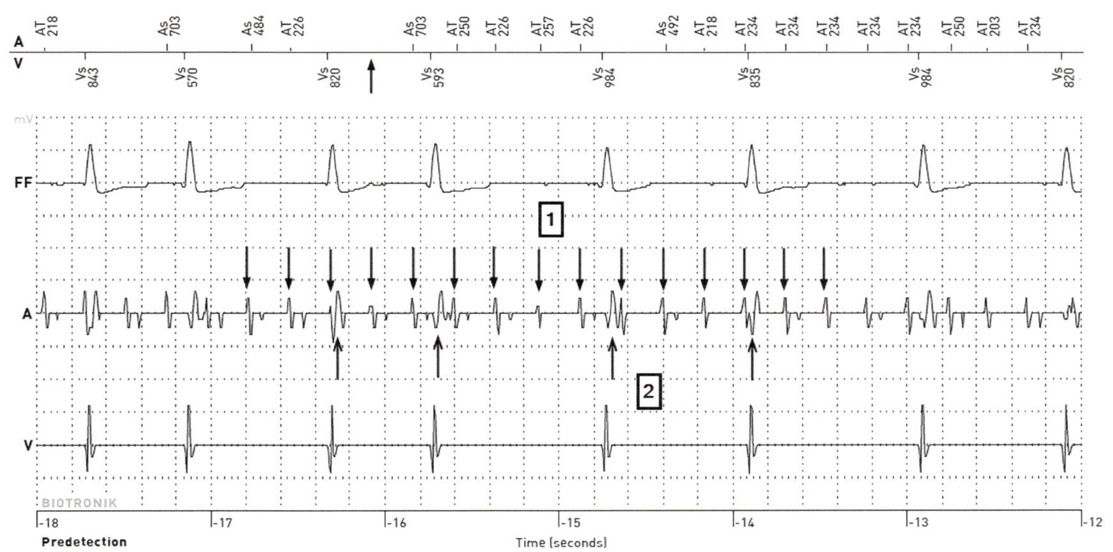

Figure 54a.

RA sensing details	
Sensing	Standard
Upper threshold [%]	---
Minimum threshold [mV]	0.3
Far-field protection after V pace [ms]	75
Far-field protection after RV sense [ms]	75
PVARP after PVC [ms]	---
PVARP after V sense	---
Atrial monitoring zone	
AT/AF zone limit [ms]	300

Figure 54b.

Figure 54a is an example of an atrial arrhythmia episode reported via routine remote monitoring. Atrial sensing and detection is programmable similar to a standard atrial lead configuration. Settings are shown in Figure 54b. The atrial EGM in Figure 54a reports an atrial tachyarrhythmia episode based on the programmed AT/AF zone limit of 300 ms. The atrial EGM shows an atrial flutter [1] at approximately 250 bpm (240 ms) (↓ denotes flutter waves). There is intermittent undersensing of flutter waves at the beginning of the EGM.

4. The far-field QRS is also apparent on the atrial EGM [2] (↑ denotes far-field QRS complexes). The atrial channel is appropriately blanked from atrial sensing falling within the far-field protection after RV sense parameter (75 ms).

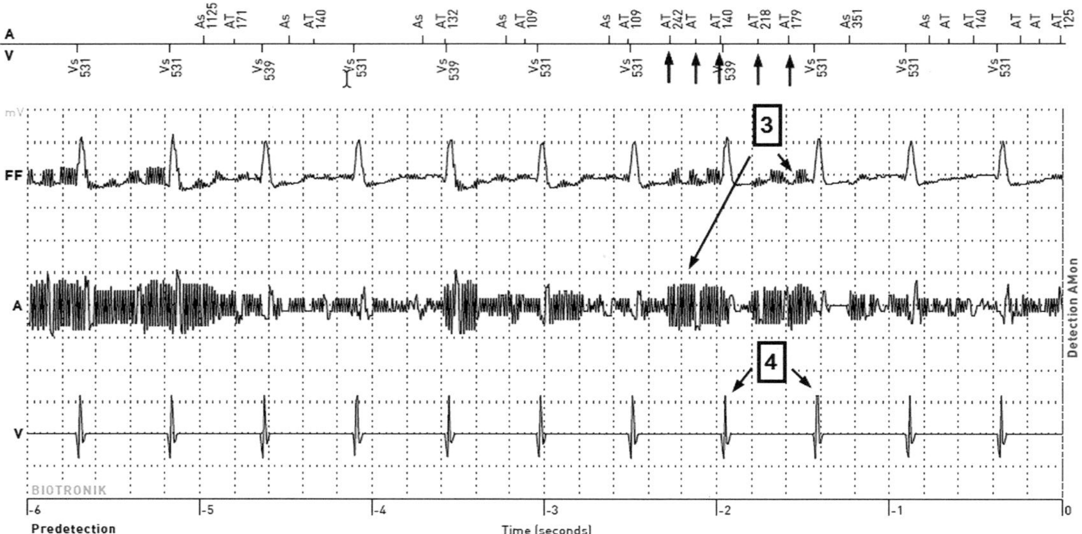

Figure 54c.

5. Figure 54c is also an example of an atrial arrhythmia episode reported via routine remote monitoring. In this case, there the atrial EGM show nonphysiologic artifact that is oversensed as an atrial arrhythmia [3]. The artifact is also apparent on the far-field EGM (RA DX ring1 to RV coil), but to a lesser extent than the atrial EGM (RA DX ring1 to RA DX ring2). The floating nature of the atrial sensing configuration makes it susceptible to unwanted external electrical signals. The high-frequency noise seen on the atrial channel and the far-field channel is likely due to EMI or myopotential oversensing.

6. The ventricular EGM shows a regular rate of approximately 100 bpm during this episode [4]. The atrial tachyarrhythmia episode reported is inappropriate.

The Biotronik DX lead feature can be very helpful in detecting atrial arrhythmias using a single RV lead. However, it also has the potential for overensing and overreporting false positives for atrial arrhythmia. This patient was brought into the clinic for further assessment, and lead testing was normal. The source of artifact was not clear and was not reproducible in the clinic.

55 | Medtronic Detection Zones with Fast VT via VT versus Fast VT via VF

DEVICE: Medtronic Claria MRI DTMA1D1 CRT-D

PATIENT: A 74-year-old male presented to the ED following an episode of ventricular tachycardia (VT) that was treated with multiple sequences of ATP and a single shock from his ICD. Upon arrival to the ED, the patient was found to be in a slow VT at 130 bpm. The patient was cardioverted with an external defibrillator and Amiodarone initiated. The patient was then transferred to the cardiac critical care unit (CCU) for further evaluation. During his stay in the CCU, the patient was in a slow VT at 140 bpm. Successful application of ATP was programmed at the bedside by the attending physician who then made permanent programming changes to the detection settings. Following these changes, the patient received a shock for a stable VT at 130 bpm. He was then seen by the device nurse specialist for final programming changes to prevent shocks for slow, stable VT.

Figures 55a, **55b**, and **55d** show the settings from pre-hospital admission, changes by the CCU physician, and final settings respectively. **Figure 55c** shows the plot graph from the episode of stable VT.

VT/VF Detection

		V. Interval (Rate)	Initial	Redetect
VF	On	300 ms (200 bpm)	18/24	12/16
FVT	OFF	250 ms (240 bpm)		
VT	On	400 ms (150 bpm)	16	12
Monitor	Monitor	500 ms (120 bpm)	20	

Detection		Rates	Therapies
AT/AF	Monitor	>171 bpm	All Rx Off
VF	On	>200 bpm	ATP During Charging, 35J x 6
FVT	OFF		(Detection is OFF) Burst(1), Ramp(1), 35J x 4
VT	On	150-200 bpm	Burst(3), 35J x 5

Enhancements On: VT Monitor, AF/Afl, Sinus Tach, TWave, Noise(Timeout)

Figure 55a.

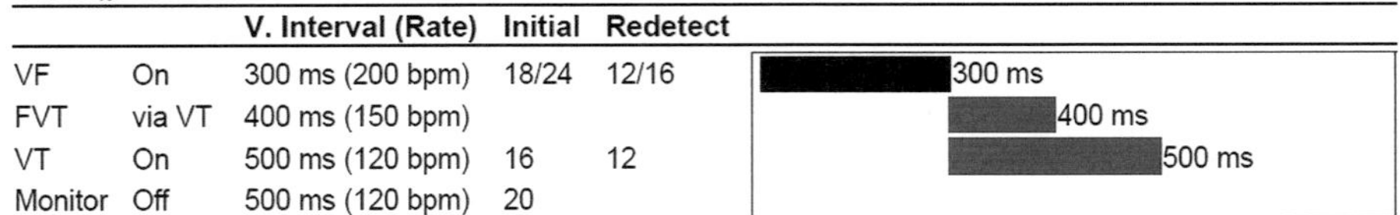

VT/VF Detection

		V. Interval (Rate)	Initial	Redetect
VF	On	300 ms (200 bpm)	18/24	12/16
FVT	via VT	400 ms (150 bpm)		
VT	On	500 ms (120 bpm)	16	12
Monitor	Off	500 ms (120 bpm)	20	

Detection		Rates	Therapies
AT/AF	Monitor	>171 bpm	All Rx Off
VF	On	>200 bpm	ATP During Charging, 35J x 6
FVT	via VT	150-200 bpm	Burst(3), 35J x 5
VT	On	120-200 bpm	Burst(3), Burst(3), some Off

Enhancements On: AF/Afl, Sinus Tach, TWave, Noise(Timeout)

Figure 55b.

Type	ATP Seq	Shocks	Success	ID#	Date	Time hh:mm	Duration hh:mm:ss	Avg bpm A/V	Max bpm A/V	Activity at Onset
VT	9	35J	Yes	633	09-Sep-2019	00:50	:01:53	48/133	---/146	Rest

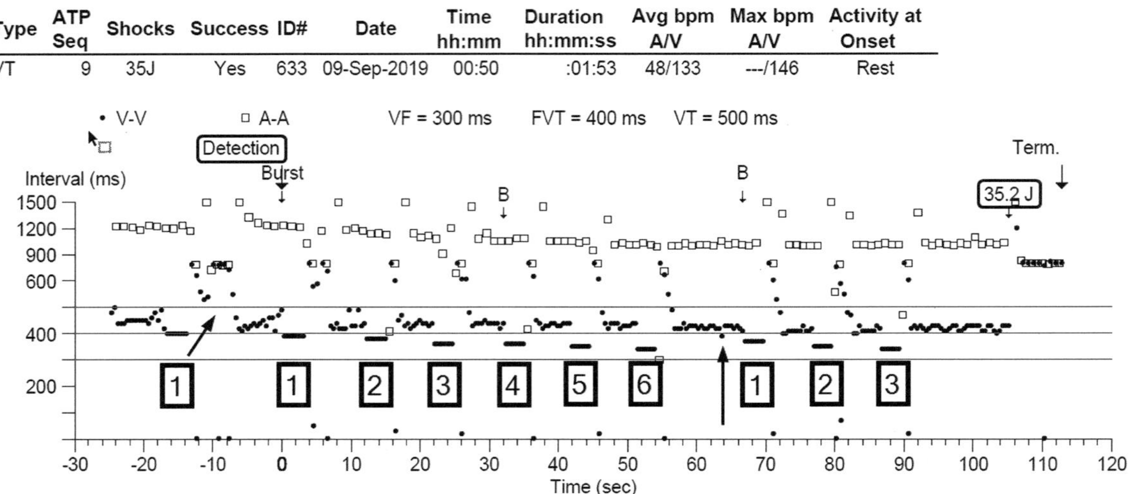

Figure 55c.

VT/VF Detection

		V. Interval (Rate)	Initial	Redetect
VF	On	400 ms (150 bpm)	18/24	12/16
FVT	via VF	300 ms (200 bpm)		
VT	On	500 ms (120 bpm)	16	12
Monitor	Off	500 ms (120 bpm)	20	

Detection		Rates	Therapies
AT/AF	Monitor	>171 bpm	All Rx Off
VF	On	>150 bpm	ATP During Charging, 35J x 6
FVT	via VF	150-200 bpm	Burst(3), 35J x 5
VT	On	120-150 bpm	Burst(3), Burst(3), Ramp(3), Ramp+(3), some Off

Enhancements On: AF/Afl, Sinus Tach, TWave, Noise(Timeout)

Figure 55d.

1. The settings in Figure 55a depict the preadmission setting: a Monitor Only zone at 120 bpm; a VT zone at 150 bpm with up to three sequences of ATP and up to five shocks; a VF zone with ATP during charging and up to six shocks. With these settings, the patient required external defibrillation to convert him out of a slow VT at a rate of 146 bpm.

2. Following the successful application of ATP, the attending CCU physician made changes to the detection settings. Figure 55b shows that the detection rate for the VT zone was reduced from 150 bpm to 120 bpm. Three additional sequences of ATP were added and the shocks removed. The purpose of these changes was to allow for numerous sequences of ATP and avoid a shock for slow, stable VT. Another change made at this time was to program the Fast VT via VT at 150 bpm with three sequences of ATP and five shocks. This zone was meant to replicate the previous VT zone. The episode depicted in the following plot graph shows an episode of stable VT that was treated with a shock despite the changes that were made to avoid shocks to a slow VT.

PLOT GRAPH ANALYSIS

1. The plot graph in Figure 55c begins with an episode of nonsustained VT that is treated with ATP and briefly interrupts the rhythm. This is denoted by the first ATP [1] and the diagonal arrow pointing toward the break in the rhythm. Detection of a new episode occurs, and we see the six sequences of ATP that are programmed in the VT zone [1-6]. None of these convert the rhythm which would have continued without further therapy; however, one interval met the FVT detection with a cycle length shorter than 400 ms (see up arrow). Because the episode has already met detection for VT and the Fast VT zone is programmed via VT, it requires only a single interval meeting the detection for Fast VT to deliver therapies programmed in the FVT zone. The next three sequences of ATP are those programmed in the FVT zone as is the ultimate 35-J shock which successfully converted the rhythm.

ANALYSIS OF FINAL SETTINGS

1. Figure 55d shows the changes that were made to prevent further shocks during a slow and stable VT. Additional attempts at ATP were added in the VT zone, including Ramp and Ramp+. More importantly, the Fast VT zone is now programmed via VF. With this change, for high-energy therapy to be delivered, the initial detection would have to be met in either the Fast VT or VF zone.

The patient underwent VT ablation. Two different VTs were ablated. He was treated with amiodarone, propranolol, and mexiletine therapy. Before hospital discharge, the patient experienced one episode of VT falling below detection at a rate of 110 bpm. He was asymptomatic and the episode self-terminated.

56 | Ventricular Tachycardia Detection and Therapy

DEVICE: Boston Scientific Dynagen EL D150 SC ICD

PATIENT: A 63-year-old patient with a history of ventricular tachycardia was implanted elsewhere with a single-chamber ICD for secondary prevention. The patient's ICD is interrogated in conjunction with an electrophysiology consultation. Consider the following episode with multiple therapies (**Figures 56a** and **56b**). Programming is shown in **Figure 56c**. Are any programming changes warranted?

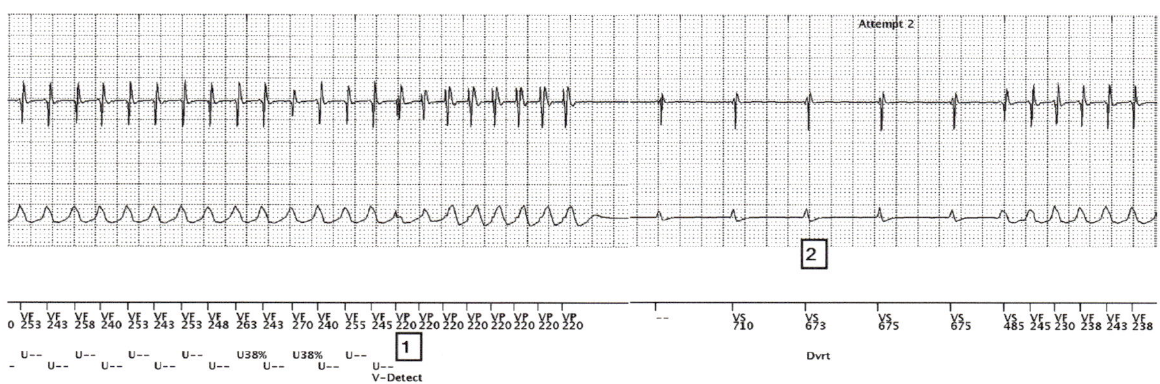

Figure 56a.

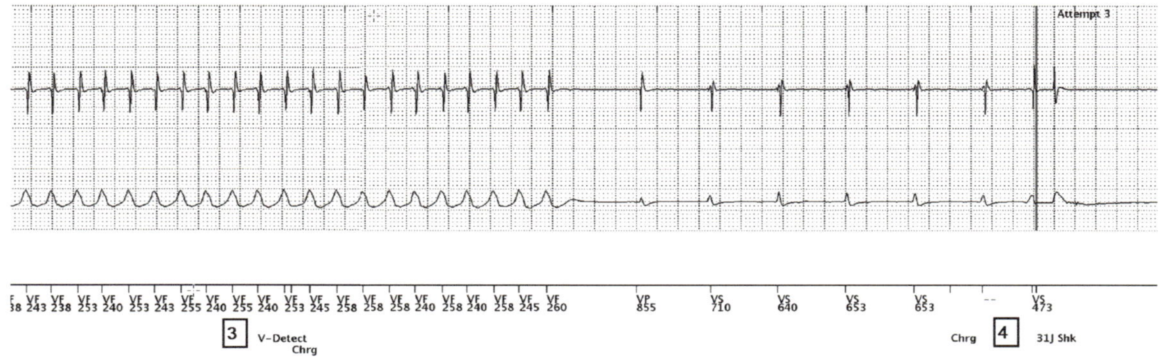

Figure 56b.

Ventricular Tachy

VF 220 bpm (273 ms)			
Detection/Redetection		**Therapy**	
Initial Duration	5.0 s	QUICK CONVERT™ ATP	On
Redetection Duration	1.0 s	Shock 1	31 J
Post-shock Duration	1.0 s	Shock 2	41 J
		Additional 41 J Shocks	6
VT 160 bpm (375 ms)			
Detection/Redetection		**ATP1**	Scan
Initial Duration	10.0 s	Number of Bursts	3
Redetection Duration	1.0 s	Pulses per Burst	
Post-shock Duration	1.0 s	Initial	10
Enhancements	Rhythm ID	Increment	0
VT Detection	On	Coupling Interval	81 %
Initial Detection	On	Decrement	10 ms
Sustained Rate Duration	03:00 mm:ss	Burst Cycle Length	81 %
Post-Shock Detection	Off	Ramp Decrement	0 ms
Rhythm ID Setup		Scan Decrement	10 ms
Passive Method	On	Minimum Interval	220 ms
Active Method	On	**ATP2**	Off
Temporary LRL	40 ppm	Number of Bursts	Off
Common Parameters		ATP Time-out	01:00 mm:ss
Stability (For Post-Shock only)	30 ms	**Shocks**	
RhythmMatch™ Threshold	94 %	Shock 1	21 J
		Shock 2	31 J
		Shock 3 -6	41 J

Figure 56c.

ANALYSIS

1. Ventricular tachyarrhythmia is detected in the VF zone [1] with intervals less than programmed VF detection of 273 ms. Quick Convert ATP is programmed on and applied by the device. The ATP successfully terminates the ventricular tachycardia. Quick Convert ATP is a Boston Scientific programming option designed to treat fast ventricular tachycardia detected in the VF zone before giving shock therapy. Quick Convert ATP delivers one burst of eight pacing pulses. It is not applied if the rate exceeds 250 bpm.

2. After the Quick Convert ATP, if two out of three intervals are slower than any detection zone [2], the shock is diverted and the episode enters redetection.

3. The ventricular tachyarrhythmia reinitiates and meets detection [3] and the device charges. The rhythm self-terminates during charging.

4. The ICD gives shock therapy during the slowed rhythm [4]. In this Boston Scientific ICD, if detection is satisfied following a diverted shock within the end-of-episode timer (10 sec) the shock is committed. This is a nonprogrammable safety feature designed to override undersensing.

CLINICAL RESPONSE

No programming changes are warranted, but other therapeutic options to control the VT were considered. The patient was started on amiodarone but because the patient has pulmonary function abnormalities, it was decided that amiodarone was not an ideal long-term solution. VT ablation was successfully accomplished.

DEVICE: Boston Scientific Energen E142 DC ICD

PATIENT: This 65-year-old male was implanted with a dual-chamber defibrillator due to a history of non-Hodgkins lymphoma and subsequent chemotherapy-induced cardiomyopathy with BiV heart failure. He also has a history of paroxysmal atrial fibrillation and severe tricuspid valve regurgitation. EGMs are shown in **Figures 57a**, **57b**, **57c**, **57d**, and **57e**. Programmed parameters are shown in **Figures 57f** and **57g**.

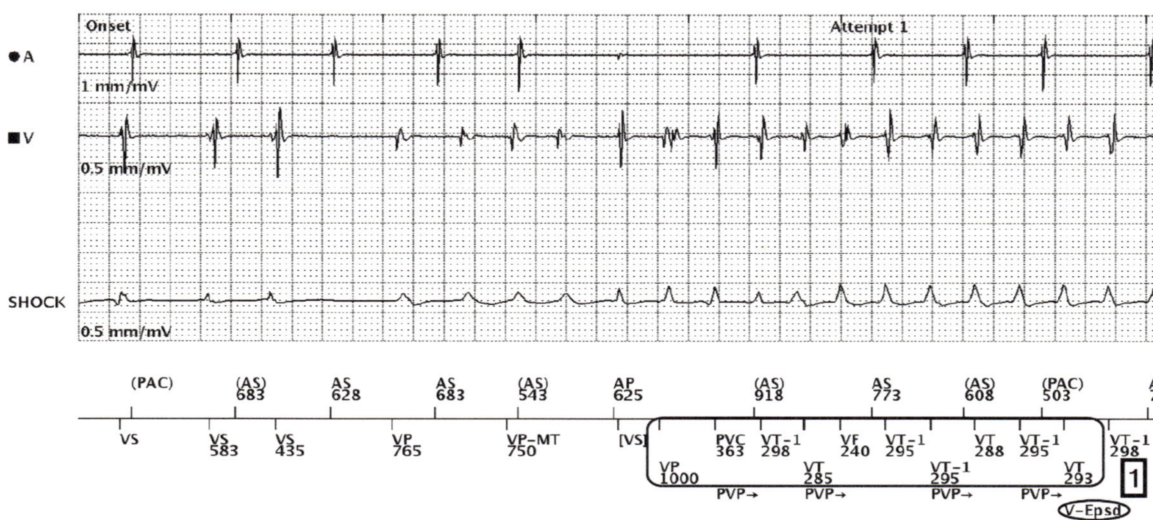

Figure 57a.

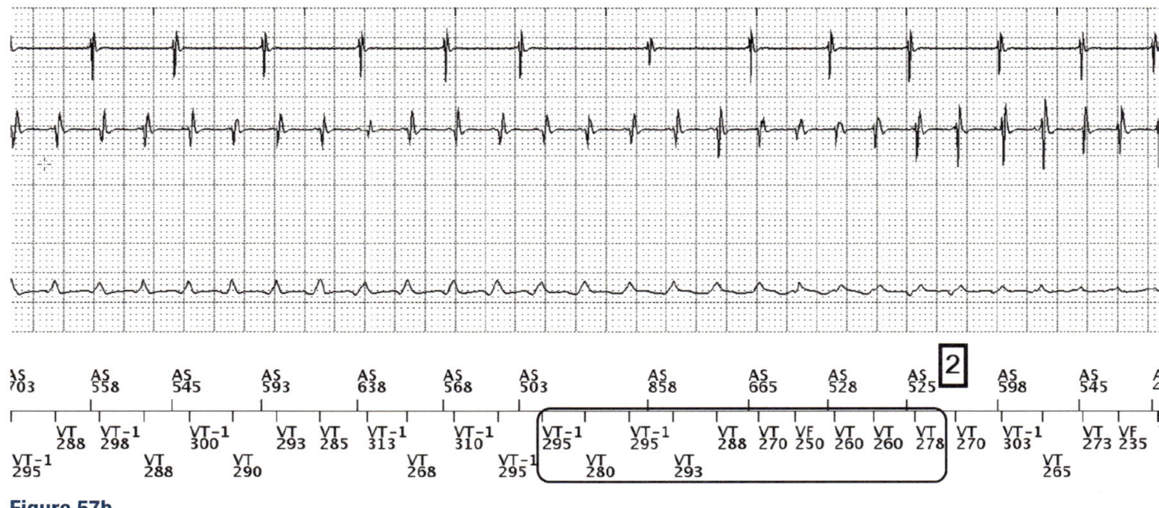

Figure 57b.

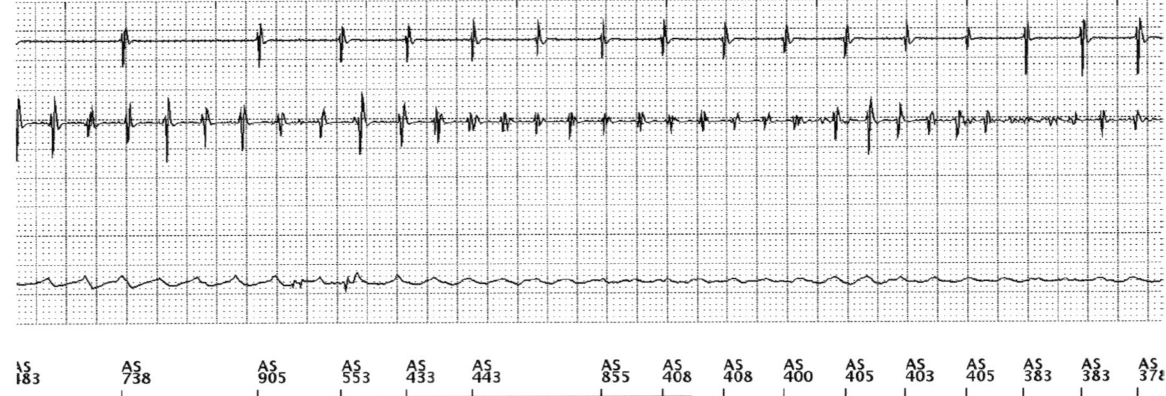

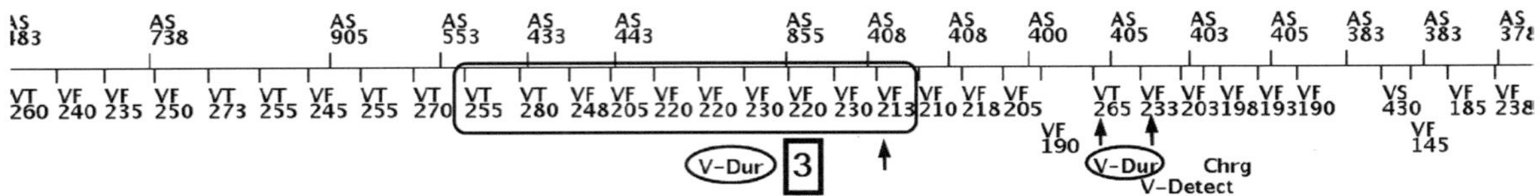

Figure 57c.

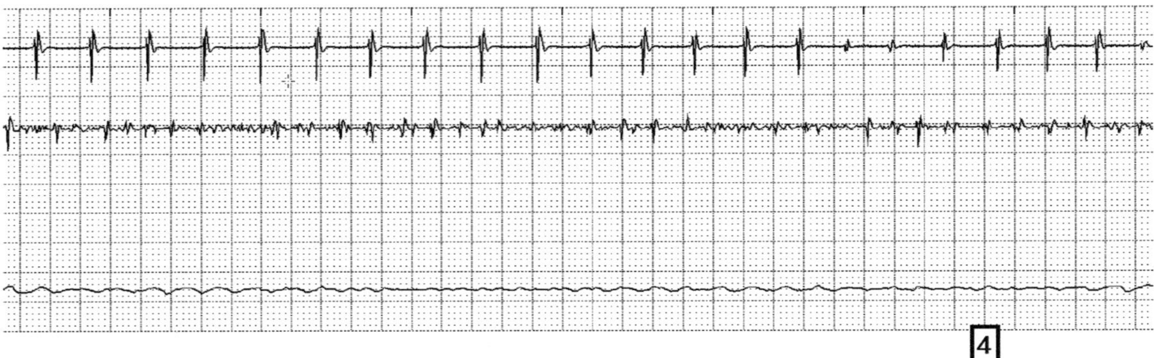

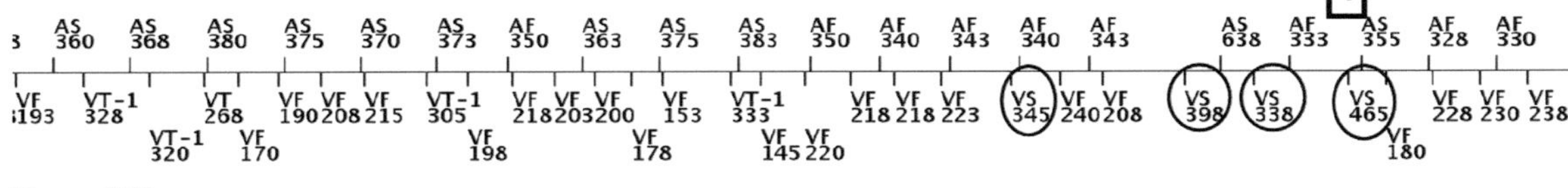

Figure 57d.

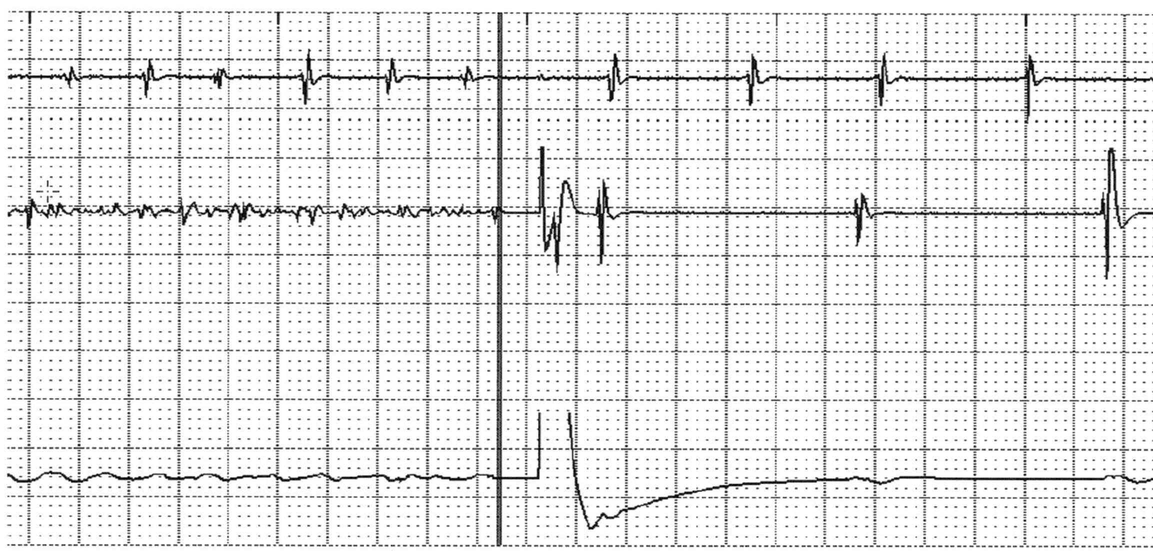

Figure 57e.

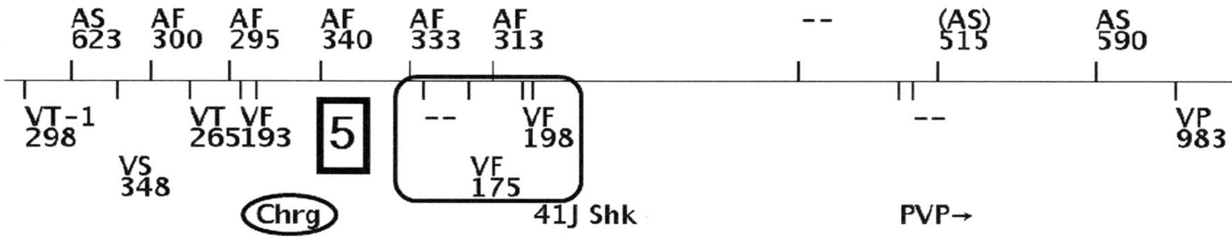

Figure 57f.

Ventricular Tachy

VF 240 bpm (250 ms)

Detection/Redetection	
Initial Duration	1.0 s
Redetection Duration	1.0 s
Post-shock Duration	1.0 s

VT 205 bpm (293 ms)

Detection/Redetection	
Initial Duration	5.0 s
Redetection Duration	1.0 s
Post-shock Duration	1.0 s
Enhancements	Rhythm ID
VT Detection	Off

Therapy	
QUICK CONVERT™ ATP	Off
Shock 1	41 J
Shock 2	41 J
Additional 41 J Shocks	6
ATP1	Burst
Number of Bursts	1
Pulses per Burst	
Initial	8
Increment	0
Coupling Interval	88 %
Burst Cycle Length	88 %
Ramp Decrement	0 ms
Minimum Interval	220 ms
ATP2	Off
Number of Bursts	Off
ATP Time-out	01:00 mm:ss
Shocks	
Shock 1	31 J
Shock 2	41 J
Shock 3 -6	41 J

Ventricular Tachy (Continued)

VT-1 180 bpm (333 ms)			**ATP1**	Scan
Detection/Redetection			Number of Bursts	3
Initial Duration	30.0 s		Pulses per Burst	
Redetection Duration	1.0 s		Initial	8
Post-shock Duration	1.0 s		Increment	1
Enhancements	Rhythm ID		Maximum	10
VT-1 Detection	On		Coupling Interval	84 %
Initial Detection	On		Decrement	6 ms
Sustained Rate Duration	Off mm:ss		Burst Cycle Length	84 %
Post-Shock Detection	Off		Ramp Decrement	0 ms
Rhythm ID Setup			Scan Decrement	6 ms
Passive Method	On		Minimum Interval	220 ms
Active Method	On		**ATP2**	Off
Temporary LRL	50 ppm		Number of Bursts	Off
Common Parameters			ATP Time-out	01:00 mm:ss
Atrial Tachy Discrimination	On		**Shocks**	
AFib Rate Threshold	170 bpm		Shock 1	21 J
Stability	20 ms		Shock 2	31 J
			Shock 3 -5	41 J
Ventricular Tachy Therapy Setup				
ATP			**Shock (All Shocks)**	
Ventricular ATP Amplitude	5.0 V		Waveform	Biphasic
Ventricular ATP Pulse Width	1.0 ms		Committed Shock	Off
Magnet and Beeper			Lead Polarity	Initial
Magnet Response	Inhibit Therapy		Shock Lead Vector	RV Coil to RA Coil
Beep During Capacitor Charge	Off			and Can

Figure 57g.

ANALYSIS

1. The defibrillator considers the onset of a probable tachyarrhythmic episode when three successive fast intervals are detected. The episode initiates and the duration timer starts when eight out of ten intervals are counted as "fast," meaning the intervals fall within any tachycardia detection zone. Each of the last eight intervals in segment [1] met this requirement and it is in the VT-1 zone that the device initiated its duration counter. In order for it to ultimately classify this episode as VT-1, no fewer than six out of every 10 intervals must be detected as fast until duration is met, in this case, 30 seconds. At that point, VT-1 associated therapies would have been initiated.

2. Although the episode began in the VT-1 zone, segment [2] shows where eight out of 10 intervals fell in the VT zone. While still counting toward VT-1 duration, the pulse generator has now started the duration counter for VT as well, in this case, 5 seconds. Thus, if no fewer than six out of every 10 intervals for the next 5 seconds are fast enough to meet the programmed VT rate criteria, then the episode will have met VT detection and duration. The episode will then be classified as VT and therapies programmed in this zone would be initiated.

3. In Figure 57c, the segmented series of 10 intervals meets the rate criteria for VF while, simultaneously, the VT 5-second duration counter has passed, denoted by "V-Dur" [3]. The first of two arrows seen in this EGM points to where the VF duration counter of 1 second has passed. However, due to the next interval falling below the VF zone and into the VT zone, the device waits for the next beat that meets VF rate criteria (second arrow) before it detected VF, denoted by "V-Detect" and, finally, charging to deliver therapy has begun which is denoted by "Chrg."

4. A Boston Scientific defibrillator will divert therapy when fewer than six fast intervals occur in a 10-interval rolling window. In Figure 57d, there are four circled VS intervals [4], which occurred due to undersensing. Had one additional slow interval occurred within the same 10-interval window, therapy would have been diverted until redetection was met again. The atrial events are also faster in the rhythm strip due to retrograde conduction or development of atrial arhythmia.

5. Following capacitor charge, there is a 135-ms refractory window in which any sensed events are ignored. The first sensed event following this window must then be denoted by two dashes rather than an identified interval because the interval is unknown [5]. With Committed Shock programmed off, see Figure 57g, the reconfirmation takes place when two of three intervals fall within a therapy zone. The shock is synchronized to the second of these and, in this case, successfully converted the arrhythmia.

CLINICAL RESPONSE

When evaluated in the clinic, it was felt that no immediate programming changes were required and observation by remote monitoring would continue. The patient was being evaluated for heart transplant but unfortunately died of progressive heart failure following a lengthy hospital stay.

58 | Defibrillator Therapy Following Episode Termination

DEVICE: Boston Scientific Dynagen Mini D022 DC ICD

PATIENT: A 55-year-old male with severe multi-vessel coronary artery disease and ischemic cardiomyopathy received an ICD following cardiac arrest secondary to ventricular fibrillation. The EGMs (**Figures 58a**, **58b**, **58c**, and **58d**) and programmed parameters (**Figure 58e**) are shown below. Why was a shock delivered in the absence of an ongoing tachyarrhythmia?

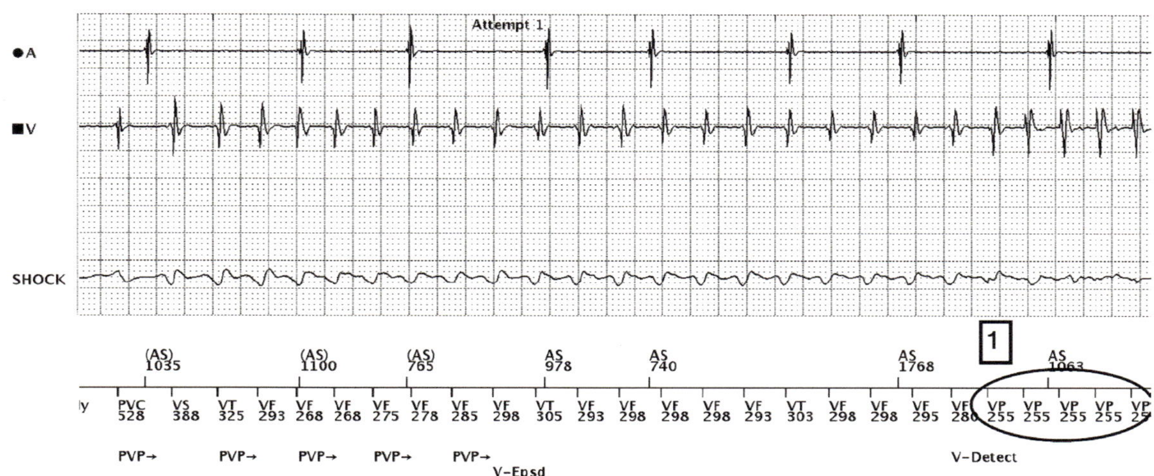

Figure 58a.

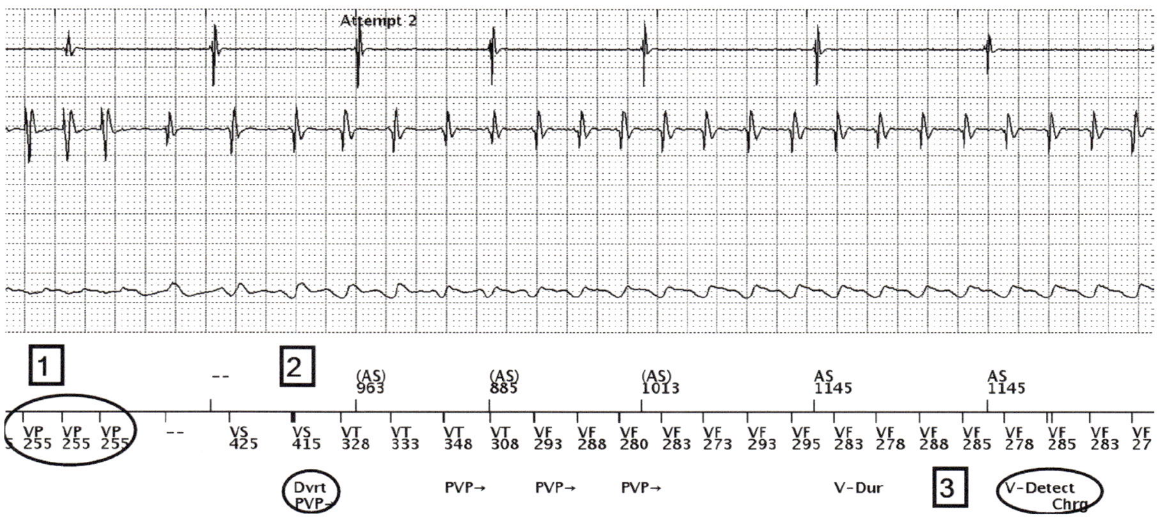

Figure 58b.

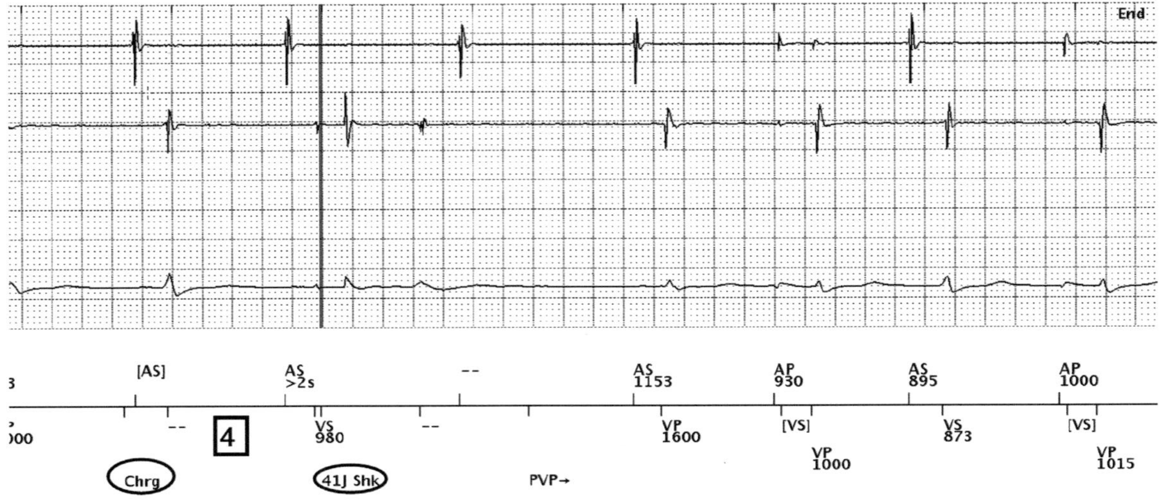

Figure 58c.

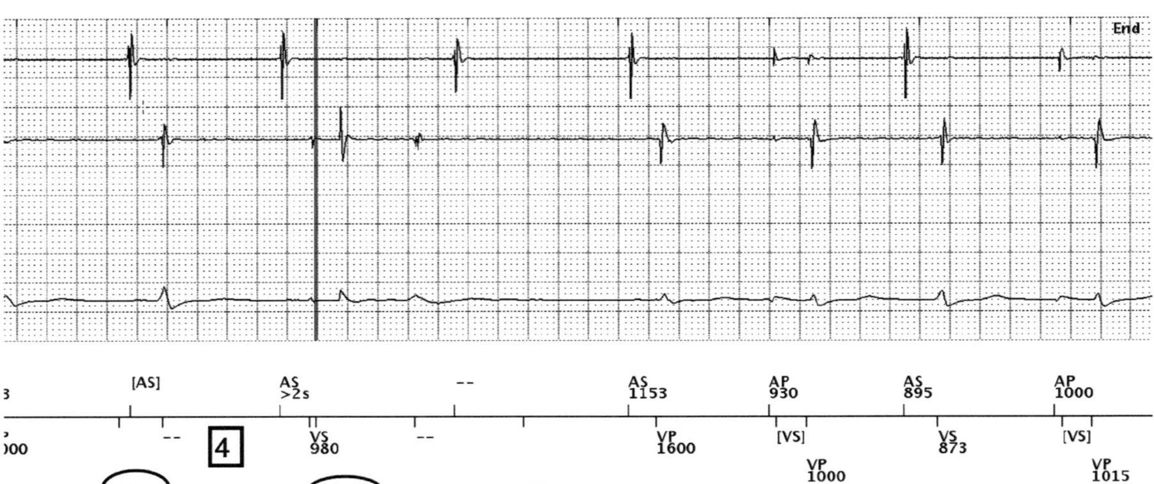

Figure 58d.

VF 200 bpm (300 ms)		Therapy	
Detection/Redetection		QUICK CONVERT™ ATP	On
Initial Duration	2.5 s	Shock 1	41 J
Redetection Duration	1.0 s	Shock 2	41 J
Post-shock Duration	1.0 s	Additional 41 J Shocks	6
VT 170 bpm (353 ms)		**ATP1**	Off
Detection/Redetection		Number of Bursts	Off
Initial Duration	10.0 s	**ATP2**	Off
Redetection Duration	1.0 s	Number of Bursts	Off
Post-shock Duration	1.0 s	**Shocks**	
		Shock 1	Off J
		Shock 2	Off J
		Shock 3 -6	Off J

Ventricular Tachy Therapy Setup			
ATP		**Shock (All Shocks)**	
Ventricular ATP Amplitude	5.0 V	Waveform	Biphasic
Ventricular ATP Pulse Width	1.0 ms	Committed Shock	Off
Magnet and Beeper		Lead Polarity	Initial
Magnet Response	Inhibit Therapy	Shock Lead Vector	RV Coil to RA Coil
Beep During Capacitor Charge	Off		and Can

Figure 58e.

VF 220 bpm (273 ms)		Therapy	
Detection/Redetection		QUICK CONVERT™ ATP	On
Initial Duration	8.0 s	Shock 1	41 J
Redetection Duration	1.0 s	Shock 2	41 J
Post-shock Duration	1.0 s	Additional 41 J Shocks	6
VT 170 bpm (353 ms)		**ATP1**	Burst
Detection/Redetection		Number of Bursts	4
Initial Duration	10.0 s	Pulses per Burst	
Redetection Duration	1.0 s	Initial	10
Post-shock Duration	1.0 s	Increment	0
Enhancements	Rhythm ID	Coupling Interval	81 %
VT Detection	On	Decrement	0 ms
Initial Detection	On	Burst Cycle Length	81 %
Sustained Rate Duration	03:00 mm:ss	Ramp Decrement	0 ms
Post-Shock Detection	Off	Scan Decrement	0 ms
Rhythm ID Setup		Minimum Interval	220 ms
Passive Method	On	**ATP2**	Burst
Active Method	On	Number of Bursts	4
Temporary LRL	60 ppm	Pulses per Burst	
Common Parameters		Initial	10
Atrial Tachy Discrimination	On	Increment	0
AFib Rate Threshold	170 bpm	Coupling Interval	81 %
Stability	20 ms	Decrement	0 ms
RhythmMatch™ Threshold	94 %	Burst Cycle Length	81 %
		Ramp Decrement	0 ms
		Scan Decrement	0 ms
		Minimum Interval	220 ms
		ATP Time-out	01:00 mm:ss
		Shocks	
		Shock 1	Off J
		Shock 2	Off J
		Shock 3 -6	Off J

Figure 58f.

ANALYSIS

1. This episode of VT began at a rate of approximately 200 bpm, meeting the rate criteria for VF, and was initially treated with a single sequence of ATP [1]. The ATP slowed, but did not convert the rhythm.

2. While the rhythm continued, the rate fell below the detection VF zone for at least two out of three beats, causing the device to divert therapy [2].

3. Several beats later the ventricular rate accelerated and met criteria for VF [3]. Having met VF detection criteria, the device began charging to deliver high-energy therapy.

4. Meanwhile, the rhythm spontaneously converted to sinus bradycardia, however, once the device charged fully, a shock was still delivered [4] despite a rhythm of sinus brady-cardia and Committed Shock being programmed OFF (see Figure 58e).

5. The shock was delivered because a Boston Scientific defibrillator will not divert two therapies in a row.

The following programming changes were made: The VT Zone Detection criteria remained unchanged; however four sequences of ATP were added with no shocks in this zone (**Figure 58f**). The VF detection rate was increased to 220 bpm and the initial duration was extended to 8 seconds. VF detection rate and duration should not be increased in patients with presyncope or lightheadedness with arrhythmias. Those patients are better served with antiarrhythmic drugs and or ablation procedures.

59 | Effective CRT

DEVICE: Medtronic Claria MRI Quad DTMA1Q1 CRT-D

PATIENT: An 84-year-old patient with nonischemic cardiomyopathy, left bundle branch block (LBBB), and heart failure has a dual-chamber ICD for primary prevention. The patient progressed to Class III NYHA functional status with an ejection fraction of 19% and LBBB with QRS duration of > 150 ms. The patient underwent an upgrade to a CRT-D device. The patient's underlying rhythm is sinus rhythm. The patient was programmed with AdaptivCRT set to Adaptive Bi-V and LV. This Medtronic CRT feature allows the device to adjust the paced and sensed AV intervals and provide adaptive LV only pacing to reduce unnecessary RV pacing. Parameters are shown in **Figure 59a**.

Parameter Summary					
Mode	DDD	Lower Rate	60 bpm	AdaptivCRT	Adaptive Bi-V and LV
Mode Switch	150 bpm	Upper Track	130 bpm	V. Pacing	LV
		Upper Sensor	120 bpm	Paced AV	140 ms
				Sensed AV	120 ms

Figure 59a.

In conjunction with AdaptivCRT, the diagnostic EffectivCRT algorithm helps evaluate the effectiveness of CRT therapy. It evaluates successful Bi-V or LV capture by morphology assessment. The basic premise is that when pacing from an electrode the activation must proceed away from the source resulting in predominantly negative QS configuration on that electrode recording. Ineffective pacing or presence of fusion will result in a positive R wave. Based on this, the EffectivCRT determines the percentage of effective CRT pacing and provides diagnostic data. At least 5 of 8 signals need to be labeled ineffective to store the diagnostic episode. Consider the data and EGM provided by the EffectivCRT diagnostic in **Figures 59b** and **59c**.

Since Last Session
01-May-2019 to 06-Aug-2019
97 days

Total VP	94.9 %
AS-VS	4.0 %
AS-VP	94.5 %
AP-VS	< 0.1%
AP-VP	1.4 %
Total VP*	94.9 %
Effective	92.8 %
Ineffective	2.1 %
VSR Pace	3.8 %
VS	1.3 %
CRT Pacing	
Bi-V	4.1 %
LV	95.9 %

Figure 59b.

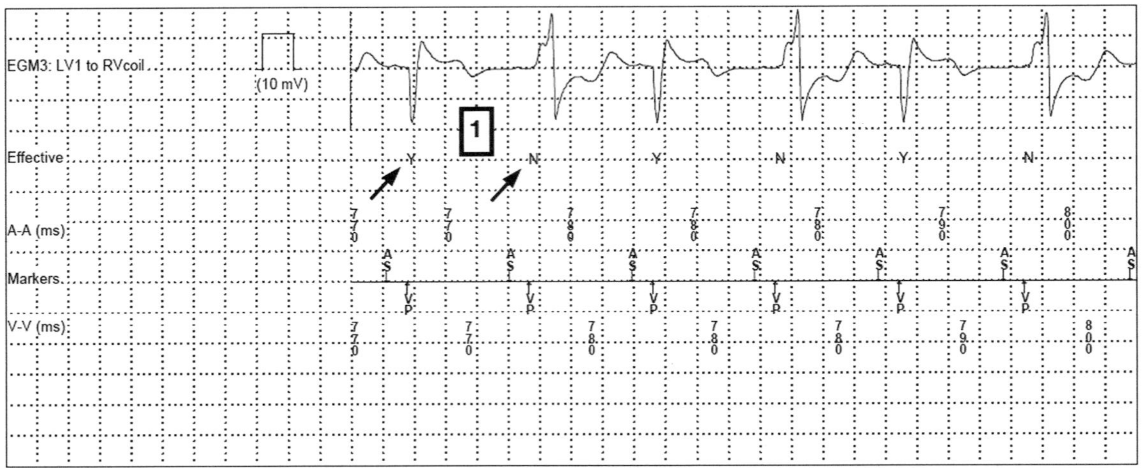

Figure 59c.

ANALYSIS

1. In this case, the AdaptivCRT feature, based on real-time intrinsic measurements and PR interval evaluation, has programmed LV only pacing with sensed AV delay of 120 ms as shown in Figure 59a. The EffectivCRT diagnostic has provided an episode with EGM strip that displays markers identifying a therapeutic LV pace with the "Y" marker and a non-therapeutic LV pace with the "N" marker [1]. This designation is device determined through an algorithm that analyzes QRS morphology. It uses the LV pace cathode to RV coil vector EGM. Further assessment is needed to determine what mechanism causes the "N" events identified by the device, and why the current CRT programmed settings may not be resulting in the most effective CRT therapy.

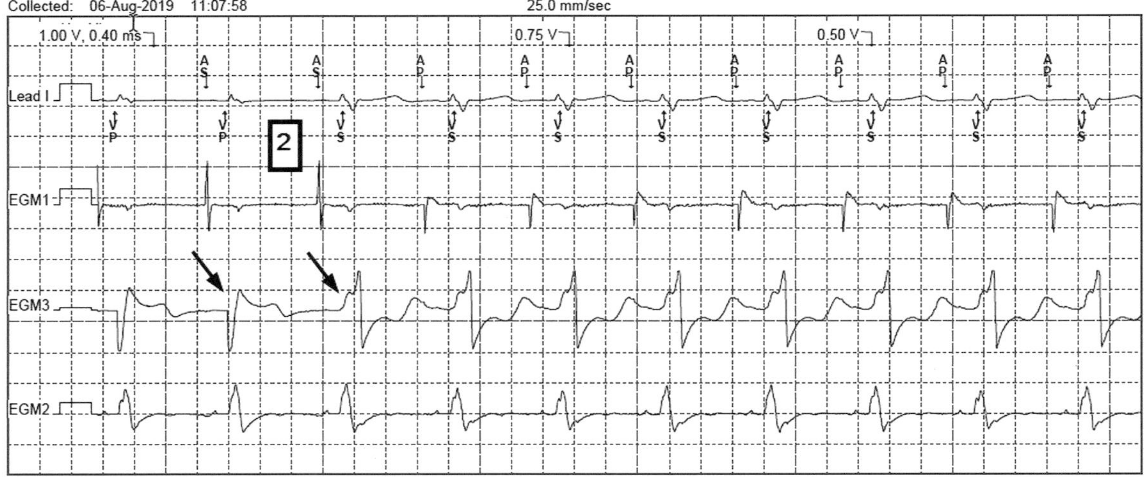

Figure 59d.

2. The EGM taken from atrial threshold testing shown in **Figure 59d** gives us the insight needed. The morphologies of LV paced and intrinsically conducted V-sensed events [2] are very similar to the events identified as ineffective LV paced events from Figure 59b. There are two scenarios that may cause this result. First is a shortened PR interval with native conduction faster than the programmed sensed AV delay. The second scenario is the loss of LV capture. If native conduction was competing with the programmed AV delay a fusion with LV pacing is more likely. Since the two morphologies match so closely, loss of LV capture is the more likely underlying cause.

Pacing Details	Atrial	RV	LV		
Amplitude	1.50 V	4.50 V	1.75 V		
Pulse Width	0.40 ms	0.40 ms	0.40 ms		
Capture Management	Adaptive	Monitor	Adaptive		
Amplitude Margin	2.0 X		+ Auto ← 3		
Min. Adapted Amplitude	1.50 V				
Max. Adapted Amplitude			6.00 V		
			Atrial(4076)	RV(6947) SVC	LV(4598)
Pacing Impedance			342 ohms	323 ohms	1121 ohms
Defibrillation Impedance				RV=45 ohms SVC=55 ohms	
Pace Polarity			Bipolar	Bipolar	LV1 to LV2
Capture Threshold			0.500 V @ 0.40 ms	2.250 V @ 0.40 ms	1.125 V @ 0.40 ms
Measured On			06-Aug-2019	06-Aug-2019	06-Aug-2019
Programmed Amplitude/Pulse Width			1.50 V / 0.40 ms	4.50 V / 0.40 ms	1.75 V / 0.40 ms

Figure 59e.

3. LV capture management is programmed on using the +Auto Amplitude Margin [3]. The LV amplitude is currently programmed 1.75 V/0.4 ms based on capture management threshold of 1.125 V/0.4 ms and +0.5 V margin (**Figure 59e**).

CLINICAL RESPONSE

The +Auto safety margin of 0.5 V may not be enough margin to cover the normal variation of LV threshold for this patient. The Auto safety margin feature was programmed off and a fixed margin of 1.0 V was programmed. The EffectivCRT diagnostic will be reassessed with the next routine remote follow-up in 3 months to verify the effective CRT pacing percentage is improved.

60 | CRT Pacing Diagnostics

DEVICE: Biotronik Ilivia 7 HF-T QP 404620 CRT-D

PATIENT: A 79-year-old patient with dilated cardiomyopathy and chronic atrial fibrillation was implanted at his local hospital with a CRT-D device. The patient is seen annually in our heart failure clinic with device interrogation at that time. Routine remote CRT-D follow-up is done at the patient's local clinic. An in-office device interrogation revealed that the CRT pacing percentage had declined significantly compared to the prior year (**Figures 60a** and **60b**). What features of this CRT-D device may help with understanding the underlying cause of the change in BiV pacing percentage?

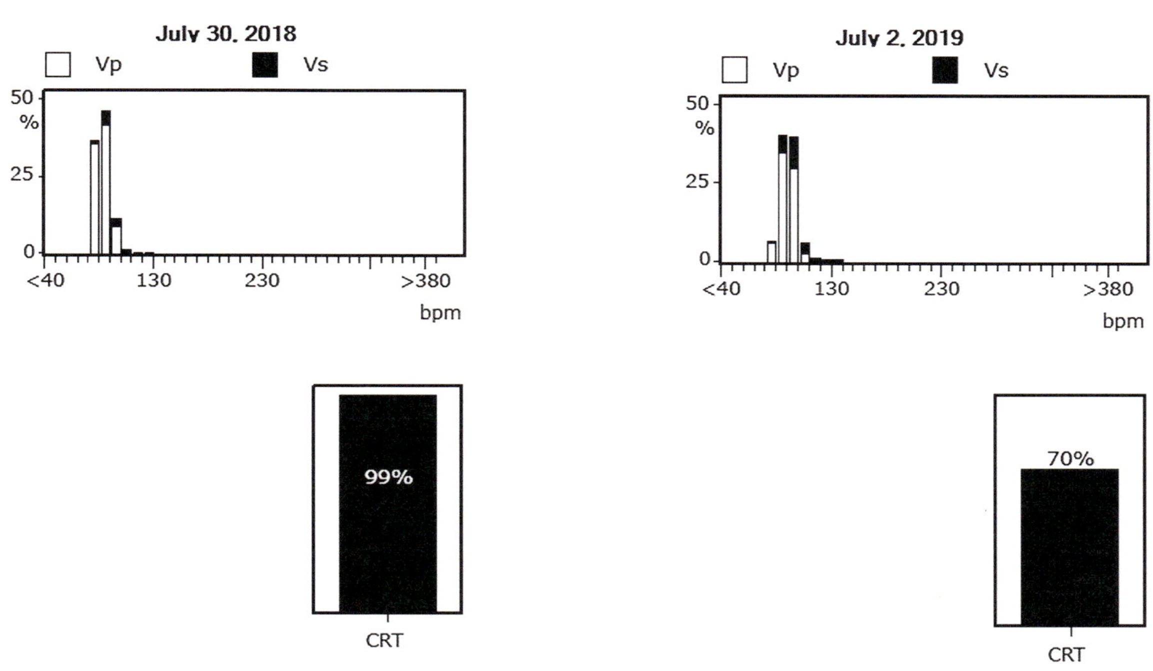

Figure 60a.

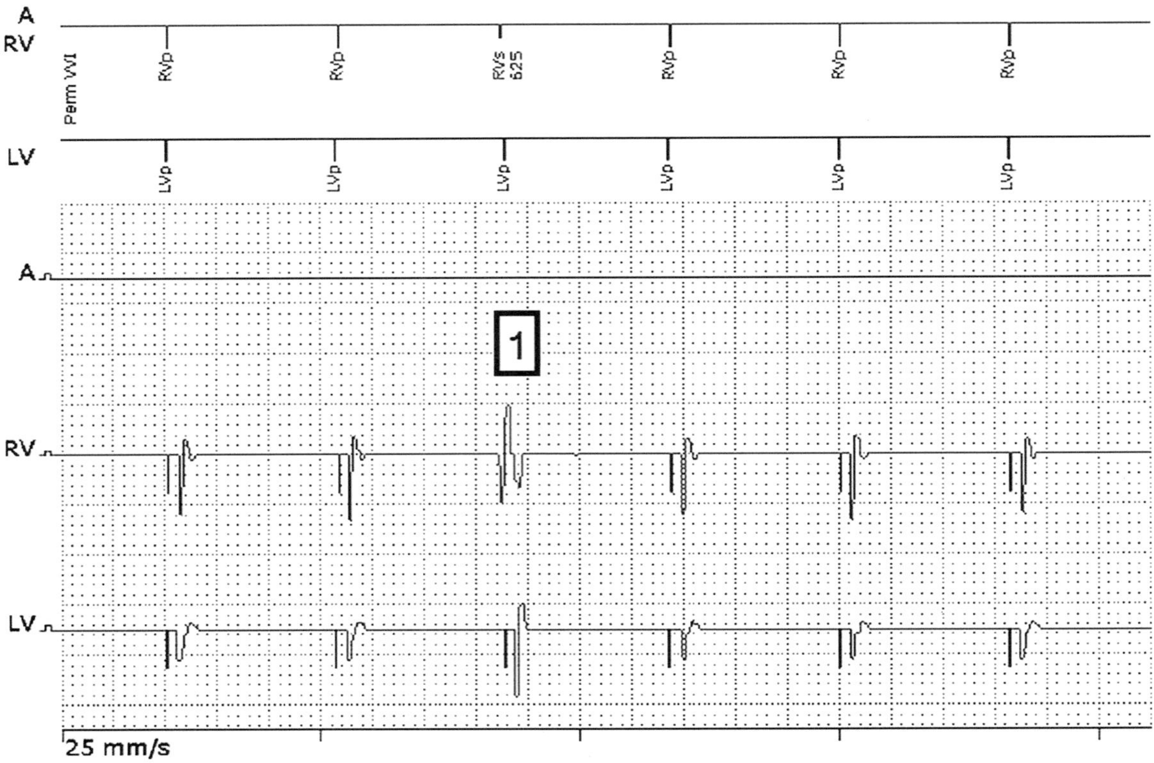

Figure 60b.

ANALYSIS

1. The presenting EGM in Figure 60b illustrates BiV pacing with one LV triggered paced (RVS with LVP) event [1]. This EGM provides some evidence of early intrinsic behavior which would detract from BiV pacing. Further investigation is needed to determine what mechanism could be causing the loss of BiV pacing.

2. This Biotronik CRT-D offers a CRT Pacing Interrupt feature. Loss of CRT pacing triggers an event with EGM recording. The loss of CRT pacing event is triggered when at least 20 of 48 ventricular events are not LV paced. **Figure 60c** includes the episode list and **Figure 60d** is one of the CRT pacing interrupt recordings.

Recordings - Episodes

No.	Time	Zone	PP [ms]	RR [ms]	Description	PP [ms]	RR [ms]
14	07/11/18 01:19	---	***	***	Periodic IEGM	***	***
13	06/10/18 00:52	---	***	***	CRT pacing interrupt	***	***
12	05/28/18 16:49	---	***	***	CRT pacing interrupt	***	***
11	05/17/18 13:38	---	***	***	CRT pacing interrupt	***	***
10	05/11/18 17:32	---	***	***	CRT pacing interrupt	***	***
9	05/09/18 00:52	---	***	***	CRT pacing interrupt	***	***

Figure 60c.

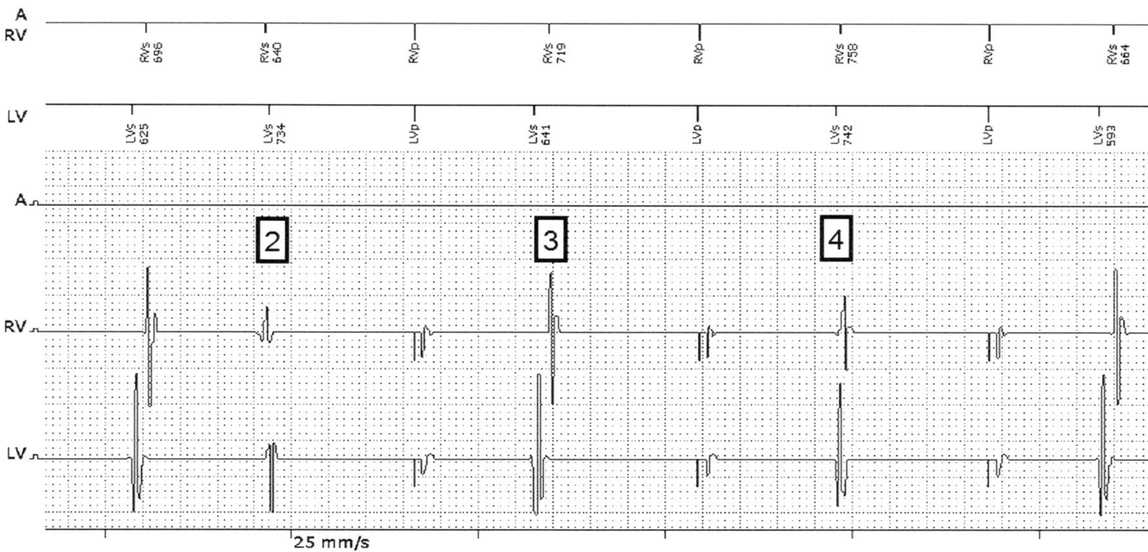

Figure 60d.

3. This EGM recording from the loss of CRT pacing feature is very informative. It demonstrates a period of 50% CRT. It includes both RV and LV EGM recordings. This reveals at least three different sensing phenomena. In the first sensed event [2] the RV sense precedes the LV sense by 94 ms. The second sensed event [3] the LV sense precedes the RV event by 105 ms, and at [4] LV precedes RV by 16 ms. The early ventricular events are likely multifactorial. The second sensed event [3] is likely left ventricular PVC with delayed conduction to the local right ventricular site.

CLINICAL RESPONSE

The patient was referred for electrophysiology consultation with Holter ECG monitor testing. Increasing the patient's lower pacing rate from 70 bpm to 80 bpm was considered, but not implemented. Medical therapy was adjusted to suppress the PVCs and to improve CRT delivery.

61 | CRT Pacing Diagnostics

DEVICE: Biotronik Ilivia 7 HF-T QP ProMRI 404621 CRT-D

PATIENT: An 86-year-old patient with heart failure, left bundle branch block and left ventricular ejection fraction of 25% was implanted with a BiV ICD (CRT-D) elsewhere. An alert remote transmission was received which demonstrated the BiV pacing percentage to have decreased from 98% to 86% within 24 hours as seen in **Figure 61a**. (EGM is shown in **Figure 61b**, programmed parameters in **Figure 61c** and rate histograms and pacing percentages in **Figure 61d**.) What information can be obtained from the EGM and what programming changes could be made to maintain higher BiV pacing percentages?

Paced rhythm		24 h	Mean values
Atrial pacing (Ap) [%]		98	88
Right ven. pacing (RVp) [%]		99	98
Left ven. pacing (LVp) [%]		86	98

Figure 61a.

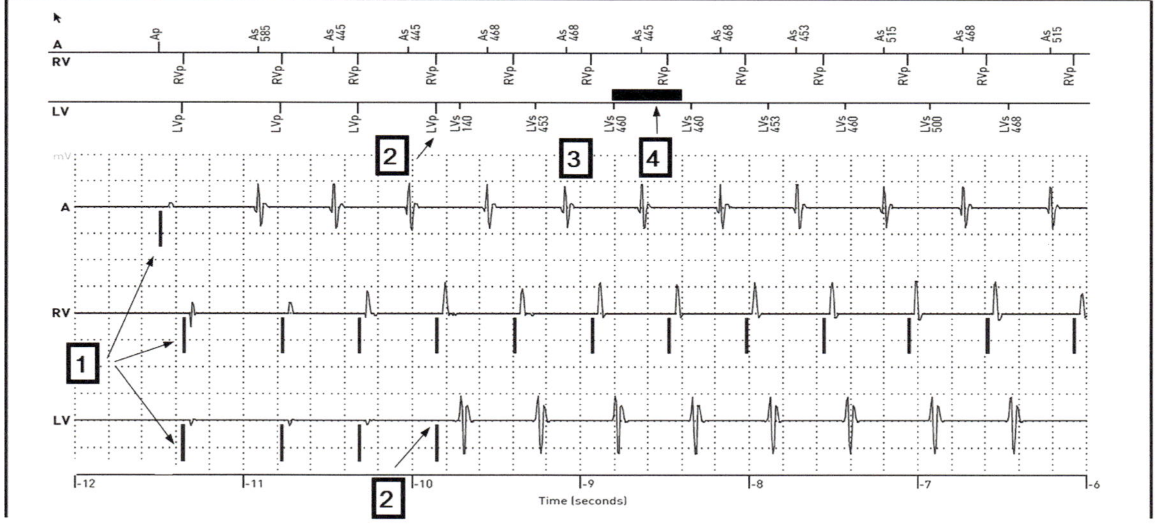

Figure 61b.

Brady basics	
Mode	DDD-CLS
Basic rate [bpm]	60
Night rate [bpm]	---
Night begins	---
Night ends	---
Rate hysteresis [bpm]	---
Rate scan	---
Upper rate [bpm]	130
Atrial upper rate [bpm]	200
PVARP [ms]	225
PVARP extension	ON
AV delay	
Dynamics	Fixed
AV delay 1	130 ms
AV delay 2	---
Sense compensation [ms]	OFF
AV delay 1 after sense	130 ms
AV delay 2 after sense	---
AV hysteresis mode	---
AV hysteresis [ms]	---
AV scan	---
CRT	
Ventricular pacing	BiV
Initially paced chamber	LV
VV delay after Vp [ms]	0
Triggering	RVs
Maximum trigger rate [bpm]	UTR + 20 bpm
LV T-wave protection	ON

Vp suppression	
Vp suppression	OFF
Suppress pacing after X consecutive Vs	---
Support pacing after X out of 8 cycles without Vs	---
Post shock	
Mode	DDI
Basic rate [bpm]	90
Ventricular pacing	BiV
Triggering	RVs
LV T-wave protection	ON
Post-shock duration	1min 0s
AV delay [ms]	140
Sensor / Rate fading	
Maximum sensor rate [bpm]	120
Sensor gain	Medium
Rate increase [bpm/cycle]	2
Rate decrease [bpm/cycle]	0.5
Sensor threshold	Medium
Rate fading	---
CLS	
CLS response	Medium
CLS resting rate control [bpm]	+20
Vp required	Yes

Figure 61c.

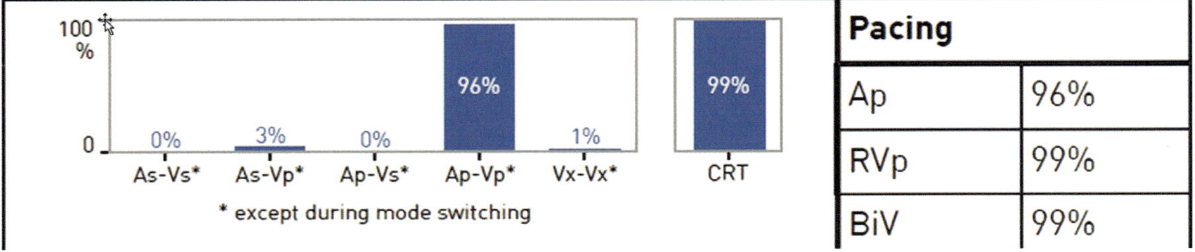

Pacing	
Ap	96%
RVp	99%
BiV	99%

Figure 61d.

ANALYSIS

1. In Figure 61b, the downward markers on CRT pacing interruption episode indicate the device delivering a pacing impulse. CRT pacing interruption episode stores an EGM, indicating there was loss of CRT pacing when there are at least 20 of 48 ventricular events that are not LV paced.

2. In Figure 61b, the first beat shows atrio-biventricular sequential pacing. The second beat is likely the start of an atrial tachycardia. The third beat shows BiV pacing via tracking. Then on the fourth beat, there is LV loss of capture [2] followed by an intrinsic LV event. The delayed event on the LV lead is due to conduction from RV pacing

3. In Figure 61b, the device is atrial sensing with RV pacing and LV sensing [3]. We also see an increase in the atrial rate when compared with the onset of the tracing.

4. Figure 61b shows that the LV-sensed event triggers the start of the LV protection window [4], which is not allowing the device to BiV pace due to the faster rate. The LV protection window serves the purpose of not allowing an LV pace to occur in the vulnerable period of repolarization that could result in a ventricular arrhythmia. Biotronik devices have the ability to sense on the LV and thus the LV-sensed event resets the maximum trigger rate and no other timing cycles. As seen in Figure 61c, the device is programmed DDD-CLS (closed loop stimulation) with a zero V-V offset along with a maximum trigger rate set to 150 bpm. When the device is programmed with CLS on, the device cannot have a V-V offset because it violates the CLS algorithm. The CLS algorithm takes eight biphasic subthreshold unipolar (tip to can) impedance measurements to assess for myocardial contractility. The first measurement happens 50 ms after the QRS and the last measurement happens 300 ms after the QRS. Turning the LV protection off could lead to the LV pacing into the vulnerable period leading to VT.

CLINICAL RESPONSE

Though the patient was not symptomatic with this CRT pacing interrupt episode the patient was brought into the clinic for programming changes. The patient performed isometric maneuvers as well as testing in multiple positions, e.g., sitting and supine, to look for LV loss of capture which could not be replicated. The maximum trigger rate (MTR) was increased to 160 bpm (400 ms) in the event the atrial rate was slower which would allow the device to BiV pace. The LV auto-capture control was changed from auto to monitor due to the fact it only runs a self-test once a day and not on a beat to beat basis. The LV amplitude was changed from 1.7 V to 2.0 V based on a measured threshold of 1.0 V at 0.4 ms. At one-month follow up the BiV pacing percentage had increased to 99% and no additional CRT Pacing Interrupt episodes as seen in Figure 61d had occurred.

Appendix A: Cases by Title

Atrial Flutter Response, Boston Scientific Ingenio K173 DC PM, Case 27 67

Atrial Loss of Capture, St. Jude Medical* Assurity DR 2240 DC PM, Case 6 13

Atrial Oversensing, Boston Scientific Punctua N051 CRT-D, Case 40 107

Atrial Oversensing with Inappropriate Mode Switch and Arrhythmia Induction,
Medtronic Advisa DR MRI A2DR01 DC PM, Case 45 117

Atrial Pacing with a Competing Junctional Rhythm, Medtronic Adapta ADDR01 DC PM, Case 3 5

Atrial Preference Pacing, Medtronic Evera XT DR DDBB1D1 DC ICD, Case 24 61

Atrial Sensed Events in Refractory Period, Medtronic Azure XT DR MRI W1DR01 DC PM, Case 15 37

Atrial Tachyarrhythmia with Atrial Intervention Pacing, Medtronic Advisa DR MRI A2DR01 DC PM, Case 28 69

Atrial Undersensing, Boston Scientific Ingenio K173 DC PM, Case 9 23

Auto-PVARP and Inappropriate Mode Switch, Medtronic Azure XT DR MRI W1DR01 DC PM, Case 32 81

Crosstalk Oversensing on Ventricular Channel with His Pace/Sense Lead in RV Port,
Medtronic Advisa DR MRI A2DR01 DC PM, Case 20 51

CRT Pacing Diagnostics, Biotronik Ilivia 7 HF-T QP 404620 CRT-D, Case 60 177

CRT Pacing Diagnostics, Biotronik Ilivia 7 HF-T QP ProMRI 404621 CRT-D, Case 61 181

DDI Pacing Mode, Boston Scientific Essentio MRI L111 DC PM, Case 13 33

Defibrillator Therapy Following Episode Termination, Boston Scientific Dynagen Mini D022 DC ICD, Case 58 169

Effective CRT, Medtronic Claria MRI Quad DTMA1Q1 CRT-D, Case 59 173

Electromagnetic Interference in ICD, Medtronic Evera XT DR DDBB1D1 DC ICD, Case 42 111

Functional Atrial Undersensing, Boston Scientific Essentio L101 DC PM, Case 10 25

Functional Ventricular Undersensing, Boston Scientific Essentio MRI EL L131 DC PM, Case 14 35

His Pacing Threshold at Implant, Medtronic Azure XT DR MRI W1DR01 DC PM, Case 19 47

Inappropriate Mode Switch, St. Jude Medical* Assurity 2240 DC PM, Case 30 73

Loss of AV Synchrony, Medtronic Evera XT DR DDBB1D4 DC ICD, Case 4 9

Loss of AV Synchrony Due to Inappropriate Mode Switch, Boston Scientific Energen N141 CRT-D, Case 31 77

Loss of Capture and Pseudofusion, Boston Scientific Essentio L101 DC PM, Case 7 17

Loss of RV and LV Capture, Medtronic Percepta Quad W4TR01 CRT-P, Case 8 21

Managed Ventricular Pacing Mode and Ventricular Arrhythmias,
Medtronic Evera XT DR DDBB1D4 DC ICD, Case 47 123

Medtronic Detection Zones with Fast VT via VT versus Fast VT via VF,
Medtronic Claria MRI DTMA1D1 CRT-D, Case 55 157

Mode Switch During VT Detection, St. Jude Medical* Quadra Assura 3369-40Q CRT-D,
St Jude Medical* Unify Assura 3357-40 CRT-D, Case 53 145

Mode Switch Termination with Failure to Establish AV Synchrony, Boston Scientific Essentio L101 DC PM, Case 29 . . . 71

Noise Oversensing, St. Jude Medical* Anthem 3210 CRT-P, Case 41 109

Pacemaker-Mediated Tachycardia, Medtronic Sensia SEDR01 DC PM, Case 33 85

Pacemaker-Mediated Tachycardia in CRT-P, Boston Scientific Valitude X4 U128 CRT-P, Case 35 91

Pacemaker-Mediated Tachycardia Intervention, Boston Scientific Essentio EL L121 DC PM, Case 34 89

Postventricular Atrial Refractory Period (PVARP) Function, Medtronic Azure XT DR MRI W1DR01 DC PM, Case 5 11

Promoting Intrinsic Ventricular Conduction, St. Jude Medical* Ellipse DR 2411-36Q DC ICD, Case 23 59

Pseudo Undersensing in Leadless Pacemaker, Medtronic Micra VR TCP MC1VR01 SC PM, Case 21 53

Pseudo-Wenckebach Upper Rate Behavior, Boston Scientific Cognis 100-D N119 CRT-D, Case 17 43

Pseudo-Wenckebach Upper Rate Behavior, Medtronic Viva Quad XT DTBA1Q1 CRT-D, Case 16 41

Pseudo-Wenckebach Upper Rate Behavior, St. Jude Medical* Allure Quadra 3242 CRT-P, Case 18 45

Rate Drop Response, Medtronic Advisa DR MRI A2DR01 DC PM, Case 25 63

Rate Smoothing, Boston Scientific Essentio EL L121 DC PM, Case 26 65

Remote Alert Follow-Up, Boston Scientific Essentio L101 DC PM, Case 22 55

Respiratory Trends and Atrial Oversensing, Boston Scientific Inogen X4 G148 CRT-D, Case 36 95

RV Lead Failure, St. Jude Medical* Fortify Assura VR 1357-40C SC ICD, Case 43 113

RV Lead Fracture, Medtronic Evera XT DR DDBB1D1 DC ICD, Case 44 115

RV Lead Integrity Warning and T-Wave Oversensing Discrimination,
    Medtronic Evera XT DR DDMB1D4 DC ICD, Case 51 137

Short-Long-Short-Induced Ventricular Tachycardia, Boston Scientific Incepta DR E163 DC ICD, Case 46 119

Signal Artifact Monitor, Boston Scientific Essentio MRI EL L131 DC PM, Case 37 97

Single-Chamber ICD with Atrial Sensing, Biotronik Lumax 740 VR-T DX SC ICD, Case 54 153

Subcutaneous ICD Oversensing, Boston Scientific Emblem A209 S-ICD, Case 52 141

T-Wave Oversensing, St Jude Medical* Unify Assura 3357-40C CRT-D, Case 50 135

Undersensing of Atrial Arrhythmia, Medtronic Claria MRI Quad DTMA1QQ CRT-D, Case 11 27

Variation in Paced QRS Morphology, St. Jude Medical* Accent DR 2110 DC PM, Case 1 1

Ventricular Noise Reversion, St. Jude Medical* Unify Assura 3357-40 CRT-D, Case 38 101

Ventricular Oversensing with RV Lead Failure, Boston Scientific Inogen EL D141 SC ICD, Case 39 105

Ventricular Pacing in the Vulnerable Period Due to Blanking and Associated Arrhythmia,
    Boston Scientific Energen DR E143 DC ICD, Case 48 127

Ventricular Pacing in the Vulnerable Period During Atrial Flutter,
    Boston Scientific Inogen X4 G148 CRT-D, Case 49 131

Ventricular Safety Pacing, Medtronic Viva XT DTBA1D1 CRT-D, Case 12 29

Ventricular Tachycardia Accelerating to Ventricular Fibrillation with Undersensing,
    Boston Scientific Energen E142 DC ICD, Case 57 163

Ventricular Tachycardia Detection and Therapy, Boston Scientific Dynagen EL D150 SC ICD, Case 56 161

Ventricular Undersensing in a Dual-Chamber Pacemaker, Medtronic Advisa DR MRI A2DR01 DC PM, Case 2 3

---

*St. Jude Medical is now Abbott.

Appendix B: Cases by Manufacturer

Biotronik Ilivia 7 HF-T QP 404620 CRT-D, CRT Pacing Diagnostics, Case 60. 177

Biotronik Ilivia 7 HF-T QP ProMRI 404621 CRT-D, CRT Pacing Diagnostics, Case 61 181

Biotronik Lumax 740 VR-T DX SC ICD, Single-Chamber ICD with Atrial Sensing, Case 54. 153

Boston Scientific Cognis 100-D N119 CRT-D, Pseudo-Wenckebach Upper Rate Behavior, Case 17 43

Boston Scientific Dynagen EL D150 SC ICD, Ventricular Tachycardia Detection and Therapy, Case 56 161

Boston Scientific Dynagen Mini D022 DC ICD, Defibrillator Therapy Following Episode Termination, Case 58 169

Boston Scientific Emblem A209 S-ICD, Subcutaneous ICD Oversensing, Case 52 141

Boston Scientific Energen DR E143 DC ICD, Ventricular Pacing in the Vulnerable Period
     Due to Blanking and Associated Arrhythmia, Case 48 127

Boston Scientific Energen E142 DC ICD, Ventricular Tachycardia Accelerating to Ventricular Fibrillation
     with Undersensing, Case 57. 163

Boston Scientific Energen N141 CRT-D, Loss of AV Synchrony Due to Inappropriate Mode Switch, Case 31 77

Boston Scientific Essentio EL L121 DC PM, Pacemaker-Mediated Tachycardia Intervention, Case 34 89

Boston Scientific Essentio EL L121 DC PM, Rate Smoothing, Case 26 65

Boston Scientific Essentio L101 DC PM, Functional Atrial Undersensing, Case 10 25

Boston Scientific Essentio L101 DC PM, Loss of Capture and Pseudofusion, Case 7. 17

Boston Scientific Essentio L101 DC PM, Mode Switch Termination with Failure to Establish AV Synchrony, Case 29 . . . 71

Boston Scientific Essentio L101 DC PM, Remote Alert Follow-Up, Case 22 55

Boston Scientific Essentio MRI EL L131 DC PM, Functional Ventricular Undersensing, Case 14 35

Boston Scientific Essentio MRI EL L131 DC PM, Signal Artifact Monitor, Case 37 97

Boston Scientific Essentio MRI L111 DC PM, DDI Pacing Mode, Case 13 33

Boston Scientific Incepta DR E163 DC ICD, Short-Long-Short-Induced Ventricular Tachycardia, Case 46 119

Boston Scientific Ingenio K173 DC PM, Atrial Flutter Response, Case 27. 67

Boston Scientific Ingenio K173 DC PM, Atrial Undersensing, Case 9 23

Boston Scientific Inogen EL D141 SC ICD, Ventricular Oversensing with RV Lead Failure, Case 39 105

Boston Scientific Inogen X4 G148 CRT-D, Respiratory Trends and Atrial Oversensing, Case 36 95

Boston Scientific Inogen X4 G148 CRT-D, Ventricular Pacing in the Vulnerable Period During Atrial Flutter, Case 49 . . 131

Boston Scientific Punctua N051 CRT-D, Atrial Oversensing, Case 40 107

Boston Scientific Valitude X4 U128 CRT-P, Pacemaker-Mediated Tachycardia in CRT-P, Case 35 91

Medtronic Adapta ADDR01 DC PM, Atrial Pacing with a Competing Junctional Rhythm, Case 3 5

Medtronic Advisa DR MRI A2DR01 DC PM, Atrial Oversensing with Inappropriate Mode Switch
     and Arrhythmia Induction, Case 45 117

Medtronic Advisa DR MRI A2DR01 DC PM, Atrial Tachyarrhythmia with Atrial Intervention Pacing, Case 28 69

Medtronic Advisa DR MRI A2DR01 DC PM, Crosstalk Oversensing on Ventricular Channel
with His Pace/Sense Lead in RV Port, Case 20 51

Medtronic Advisa DR MRI A2DR01 DC PM, Rate Drop Response, Case 25 63

Medtronic Advisa DR MRI A2DR01 DC PM, Ventricular Undersensing in a Dual-Chamber Pacemaker, Case 2 3

Medtronic Azure XT DR MRI W1DR01 DC PM, Atrial Sensed Events in Refractory Period, Case 15 37

Medtronic Azure XT DR MRI W1DR01 DC PM, Auto-PVARP and Inappropriate Mode Switch, Case 32 81

Medtronic Azure XT DR MRI W1DR01 DC PM, His Pacing Threshold at Implant, Case 19. 47

Medtronic Azure XT DR MRI W1DR01 DC PM, Postventricular Atrial Refractory Period (PVARP) Function, Case 5 11

Medtronic Claria MRI DTMA1D1 CRT-D, Medtronic Detection Zones
with Fast VT via VT versus Fast VT via VF, Case 55 157

Medtronic Claria MRI Quad DTMA1Q1 CRT-D, Effective CRT, Case 59 173

Medtronic Claria MRI Quad DTMA1QQ CRT-D, Undersensing of Atrial Arrhythmia, Case 11 27

Medtronic Evera XT DR DDBB1D1 DC ICD, Atrial Preference Pacing, Case 24 61

Medtronic Evera XT DR DDBB1D1 DC ICD, Electromagnetic Interference in ICD, Case 42. 111

Medtronic Evera XT DR DDBB1D1 DC ICD, RV Lead Fracture, Case 44 115

Medtronic Evera XT DR DDBB1D4 DC ICD, Loss of AV Synchrony, Case 4 9

Medtronic Evera XT DR DDBB1D4 DC ICD, Managed Ventricular Pacing Mode
and Ventricular Arrhythmias, Case 47 123

Medtronic Evera XT DR DDMB1D4 DC ICD, RV Lead Integrity Warning
and T-Wave Oversensing Discrimination, Case 51 137

Medtronic Micra VR TCP MC1VR01 SC PM, Pseudo Undersensing in Leadless Pacemaker, Case 21 53

Medtronic Percepta Quad W4TR01 CRT-P, Loss of RV and LV Capture, Case 8, ... 21

Medtronic Sensia SEDR01 DC PM, Pacemaker-Mediated Tachycardia, Case 33 85

Medtronic Viva Quad XT DTBA1Q1 CRT-D, Pseudo-Wenckebach Upper Rate Behavior, Case 16 41

Medtronic Viva XT DTBA1D1 CRT-D, Ventricular Safety Pacing, Case 12. 29

St Jude Medical* Accent DR 2110 DC PM, Variation in Paced QRS Morphology, Case 1 1

St Jude Medical* Allure Quadra 3242 CRT-P, Pseudo-Wenckebach Upper Rate Behavior, Case 18 45

St Jude Medical* Anthem 3210 CRT-P, Noise Oversensing, Case 41 109

St Jude Medical* Assurity 2240 DC PM, Inappropriate Mode Switch, Case 30 73

St Jude Medical* Assurity DR 2240 DC PM, Atrial Loss of Capture, Case 6 13

St Jude Medical* Ellipse DR 2411-36Q DC ICD, Promoting Intrinsic Ventricular Conduction, Case 23 59

St Jude Medical* Fortify Assura VR 1357-40C SC ICD, RV Lead Failure, Case 43 113

St Jude Medical* Quadra Assura 3369-40Q CRT-D, Mode Switch During VT Detection, Case 53 145

St Jude Medical* Unify Assura 3357-40 CRT-D, Mode Switch During VT Detection, Case 53 148

St Jude Medical* Unify Assura 3357-40 CRT-D, Ventricular Noise Reversion, Case 38 101

St Jude Medical* Unify Assura 3357-40C CRT-D, T-Wave Oversensing, Case 50. 135

---

*St. Jude Medical is now Abbott.

Made in the USA
Monee, IL
07 July 2026

56546639R00121